Dodging Dandelions

Dodging Dandelions

A Memoir of
Love, Loss, and Acceptance

Ron Richards

Dodging Dandelions
by Ron Richards

This publication is designed to provide accurate and authoritative
information with regard to the subject matter covered. It is sold
with the understanding that the author is not engaged in
rendering professional advice. If medical advice or other
expert assistance is required, the services of a competent
professional person should be sought.

Dodging Dandelions

ISBN: 978-0-9899144-0-6 (print)
ISBN: 978-0-9899144-1-3 (e-book)
LCCN: 2013920194

Published by Mitchell Canyon Communications

Ron Richards
www.dodgingdandelions.com
ron.richards@dodgingdandelions.com

Book and Cover Design by:
Nick Zelinger, NZ Graphics
www.nzgraphics.com

Manuscript edited by:
Melanie Mulhall, Dragonheart Writing and Editing
www.DragonheartWritingandEditing.com

First Edition

Printed in the United States of America

To all those who selflessly serve as a caregiver to a loved one. Your sacrifice, love and devotion make life better for all of us.

INTRODUCTION

Sara and I were sitting in the den of our comfortable colonial home in the Detroit suburbs when she turned to me and gave me an assignment.

"We have a great story to tell, you know. It will help people understand that living with adversity doesn't have to bring you down. We've had so many wonderful adventures, despite the challenges and issues we've faced. People need to know that. We have to help them understand that living with those challenges doesn't mean you have to lead a life filled with negativity. I have no doubt that you're the best person to tell our story."

That conversation in early 2004 served as the inspiration for *Dodging Dandelions*.

Bringing this story to life took several years. I guess it isn't surprising that, at times, I struggled to will my fingers to type the words on my computer screen. When you lose the person you have loved for more than half your life, recounting it often comes slowly and with difficulty.

Sara was a fabulous woman—selfless and emotionally intelligent. Her primary purpose in life was to help others. As her breast cancer worsened, she never wavered in her insistence upon "being the best patient I can be." That phrase exemplified the upbeat approach she exhibited as she dealt with her plight. It is an approach few people could—or would—replicate. I'm convinced that it extended her life by more than a year. It was one of many lessons I learned from her as we traversed the many adventures of our life together.

A significant part of our story includes navigating the peaks and valleys of mental illness. Our daughter, Jennifer, came to us from Korea at five months old. While we were pleased to have a second child, very early on we recognized the challenges she—and we—faced. As her life has played out, she has received a variety of diagnoses. That continues to this day.

Much of her life, she has been labeled with bipolar disorder. As I was completing *Dodging Dandelions*, she received yet another diagnosis: borderline personality disorder. It seems this actually fits her best. The one thing I have learned, though, is that psychiatry is as much art as it is science. That being the case, I suspect her "label" may change again. Regardless, the issues she faces are, at times, monumental, and have had major implications for her in life. One final note—in deference to my daughter's desire to maintain her privacy, I have changed her name in the book.

As for my son, Andrew, I admire his ability to persevere. His calm and steady demeanor has regularly provided a welcome respite from the swirling drama that seemed to consume our family. Underneath it all, he cares deeply and would do anything to lend a helping hand.

Some might say that *Dodging Dandelions* is a story about adversities and how a family overcame them. I would counter by saying it's a story of determination, inspiration, doing the right thing, and most importantly, staying positive. That is my wish for you as you traverse your own adventures in life. It would be Sara's wish, too.

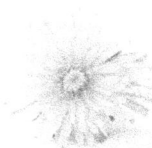

CHAPTER

1

I looked around the room. Tired, worried, and scared faces housed eyes that were searching for answers.

This was our initial visit to meet this doctor. Despite that, like us, most had probably been here before—many times. As I scanned the room I could see that the people in it were, generally, older than Sara and me. I could guess that almost everyone dreaded coming to this place. Waiting to see the doctor.

The *specialist*.

The *oncologist*.

The person who supposedly—and hopefully—had "the answer."

Sara looked up from the magazine she had been perusing and smiled, clearly happy to see me. "Where have you been?" she asked as she patted the seat of the small bench, directing me to sit next to her. Many years of marriage led me to believe that this was more idle question than real inquiry.

"Sorry. Did they give you any sense of how long it will be?"

"It shouldn't be much longer," she said, her pretty brown eyes flashing as she grabbed my hand. I could feel the apprehension flowing from her body. It created a palpable tension, one that could quickly close in on you.

I'd slipped out of a work meeting and sped along the highway paralleling Lake Michigan to make this appointment with her. The sun glistening on the small waves that broke near the lakefront on this July 1989 day made the eventual dip into the hospital parking garage's enveloping darkness a little unsettling. Sara's apprehension was capable of swallowing me up in an almost equivalent way, but I'd already had enough practice at maintaining at least a modicum of equanimity that I managed to remain calm.

"So, this doc is one that was recommended?" I asked. I actually knew but was searching for something to break the silence.

"Yes, he's supposed to be quite good," Sara replied.

Another physician on what was a growing list of cancer doctors who were doing their best to help my young wife avoid the ravages of the miserable disease.

"Sara Richards?" came the call from a middle-aged nurse.

We stood and shuffled out of the waiting room, walked down a short hallway, and went into a small exam room. The window offered a view of the glistening blue waters of Lake Michigan, where I watched the high crest of the water on the horizon. Sara was more focused on the task at hand. She knew the routine and began to unbutton her blouse as the nurse looked over her chart. She asked a few questions and then reached for a light blue hospital gown.

It wasn't too long before the doctor appeared. He introduced himself and extended his hand to Sara. He then turned, offered his hand, and said hello to me. I made a mental note of how young he looked but his credentials were impressive and he came highly recommended by Sara's former doctors in Denver. We were prepared to make him her oncologist in Milwaukee.

He initiated his exam, making small talk about our move back to the Midwest from Denver. He probed and poked around the right side of Sara's chest. The scar left from her mastectomy six years before had long ago lost its bright red color. He felt around her armpits and then her lower abdomen as he searched for something that we hoped he would not find—signs of another tumor.

"So you had radiation and hyperthermia (treatments) in Denver?" he asked, looking to Sara for confirmation of the information he was paging through on her chart. "That was in April?" he said.

Sara nodded and I could see she was getting the impatient look that meant it was close to time for her to cut to the chase. "So what do you think? What are you thinking we should do next?" she asked, her voice firm but appropriately inquisitive.

"Let me finish my exam and then we'll talk," he said, a small smile curling up the corners of his mouth as he continued his probing. His calm demeanor was clearly a significant part of his thoughtful approach. He soon finished, stepped back, and looked at the chart.

"You want answers and I understand," he said. "You have been through a lot for a woman as young as you are. You want me to offer some immediate guidance and I understand that, too. In reviewing your case, I believe we have three directions we can consider."

"As I suspect your doctors in Denver told you, we can do chemotherapy. It is the most conservative and traditional course. Second, you can do nothing. That is a viable alternative, although I don't recommend it."

"So what *do* you recommend?" I said, looking forward to hearing something we hadn't heard before.

Sara quickly spoke up. "As you get to know me, you'll learn I have lots of questions. My job is to be the very best patient I can be. I will always be cooperative and will try to keep a positive attitude. And I generally do. All I ask is that you be honest and up-front with us. I don't want any kind of runaround. Honestly, I may not have time for it. We can handle what you have to say. Just tell us what we're faced with. We'll cope."

The young doctor smiled. "I like you already," he said as his smile spread across his face.

Sara was doing what she did so well with just about everyone she met—making a meaningful connection. It was obvious he appreciated her straightforward approach.

"I saw a note somewhere in your chart that you are an occupational therapist. So your willingness to advocate for yourself is something I am not surprised to discover. I assure you, I will always be forthright with you, and I certainly won't hide anything from you."

"Okay. That's great to hear and I truly appreciate it," Sara said as she tried to keep him moving along. After a brief pause, she continued. "So what do you recommend?"

He smiled again, this time very broadly.

"The third option is this. There is a drug that recently came out of clinical trials that I believe could make a significant difference for you. The University of Wisconsin was a key site for the trials and I'm confident you are a good candidate for it. The drug is called tamoxifen. It has properties that seem to make it a very strong fighter of breast cancer. We can start it right away if you agree that it is the way to go. All the indications are that with your type of cancer and your history, this could be a good course of treatment."

"How's it administered? Is it given like chemo?" Sara asked. She despised the thought of chemotherapy. She always said it could be the last resort in fighting her disease.

"No, it comes in pill form. You take it just once daily," he said.

Sara looked my way, wanting me to offer assurance that this would make it all okay. Of course we both knew that there were no guarantees. The tamoxifen course of treatment sounded good. Sara's oncologist in Denver had been pressuring her to start chemo and she really wanted to exhaust all other options before resorting to it.

"I would like to read up on this. It sounds almost too good to be true," she said with a weak smile. As was often the case as our life had unfolded, it seemed there was now another good reason we had moved to Wisconsin. "If I can do this and avoid chemo, I'm all for it. And if it's as it sounds, I'm for going ahead with it."

The uncertainties of cancer wear heavily on everyone involved. You always want answers, even though you learn that they generally cannot be given. But you have to ask.

I broke the brief silence that had fallen on the small exam room.

"So, after reviewing Sara's case, what is your prognosis?" I said.

Our experience with our oncology docs led me to expect pretty much a canned response. The physician hesitated, but only for a moment.

"I've seen a few cases like yours, but I have to say they are relatively rare. The onset of your disease came at quite a young age. Of course, there are no certainties when you are dealing with cancer.

"In cases like yours, I like to use my dandelion example.

"Just imagine you have a beautiful home with an immaculate yard—not a blade of grass out of place. A vast expanse of nothing but green. All is going along well until, one day, you look out on the yard and out of nowhere, you see a dandelion, it's stark yellowness a nasty surprise. You have a few options.

"You can do nothing, letting it, and future dandelions, take over. You can get a tool and dig it out. Or you can use chemicals to eliminate it. In most cases, if you use either of the final two options, that dandelion will shrivel up and go away.

"But chances are," he continued, "as time goes by, more dandelions will appear. You can do all you can to avoid them. You manage them as best you can while hoping to keep them in check. What you want to avoid is having them take over. I think we can keep them under control. But, with your history, I would be surprised if you weren't always fighting off dandelions."

He paused just for a moment to let it sink in.

"You wanted me to be honest and forthright. I trust I have not been too blunt."

It was a simple, yet poignant, assessment. We appreciated his honesty.

"Thank you for being so upfront with us," Sara said, her weak smile reappearing. "I'm sure you know that we would like to hear something different. But I wouldn't be truthful if

I said we expected something different. I'll do some reading about tamoxifen and, if it's as good as it sounds, I think I'll want to start this new drug and see how it goes."

We walked to the parking lot together, holding hands and contemplating what we had just heard. "It sounds like a good drug and a good option for us to take," I said as we left the warmth of the bright sunlight and shivered as we entered the darkness and cold of the concrete parking structure.

"We'll see," said Sara with a sigh. "I like the fact I wouldn't have to do chemo. I guess when you think about it, there really isn't much to lose by doing this."

"And maybe it will keep away the dandelions," I added with a smile on my face.

"Yeah. Let's hope so," she said.

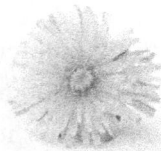

CHAPTER

2

Dealing with the sobering decisions that come with breast cancer is very different than the relatively carefree lives we had as teenagers growing up in a sleepy, northwest Ohio town.

Sara and I were fourteen when I knocked on the door of the Schroeder farmhouse to pick her up for our first date in 1966. I was taking her to a high school dance, though it would be more accurate to say that my mother was driving the two of us to the dance, since I was still too young for a license.

The dance was a pretty typical event of its time. Someone spun 45s of the Rolling Stones, Beatles, and Temptations. The girls loved to dance to every song. Most guys felt self-conscious "fast dancing" but could fumble their way through a slow dance. I fancied myself as a decent dancer, either fast or slow.

That date was the beginning of a life together that would spin and twist, rise and fall, often at precipitous speed—a ride that often made the roller coasters at nearby Cedar Point Amusement Park look tame. But it's a ride we never would have traded, despite having to deal with the stress and strain that cancer brings with it.

No man expects to make an ordinary call home when he's on the road and receive the news that his wife has cancer. Even though we had been monitoring a lump for several months, I didn't expect that news that Friday night in 1983.

I was in Canada, in the town of Bowmanville, about an hour east of Toronto. As public relations manager for the Sports Car Club of America's professional auto racing series, I assisted local race event organizers with the media. The event on this weekend was at Mosport Park. I'd spent Thursday talking up the weekend with media and wrapping up operational loose ends. Friday came and the thunderous racecars sped around the circuit. The day went routinely and, more importantly, there were no serious incidents on the course.

That evening, I went to dinner with some colleagues and returned to my modest hotel room about 11:00 p.m. My thoughts throughout dinner often wandered to Sara, and I was anxious to check in with her back in the Denver suburbs. I spent many nights on the road, and the nightly ritual of calling home was an important thread in staying connected to my wife and family.

As soon as Sara answered the phone, I knew there was something wrong. The normal bounce in her voice was absent.

At the start of the year, we discovered a lump in her right breast. It was a concern from that moment on and I nudged her to get to the doctor for an examination. She did in mid-January, and our physician assured her it was not a danger, but something to keep an eye on.

Over the next few months, we watched the lump. By May, it had grown and changed. After another doctor visit, our physician asked Sara to make an appointment with a surgeon. He'd done a needle biopsy earlier that week and said the results would be available Friday. I figured, as would most young adults, that the tumor would be benign.

Denial. So often we deal with problems or trauma in our lives in just that way. Sometimes it is an effective way to manage stress. If you're not careful, though, it can cost you your life.

I was holding the phone's handset tight to my ear. Sara burst into tears. She didn't have to tell me what I was about to hear. I already knew. Cancer had become the latest addition to the Richards family, a visitor we never anticipated, especially in the thirty-first year of Sara's life.

My mind flashed to our first date, that night in the backseat of the station wagon. How I had disliked the fact that my mother had to drive us on our date. But on that night, there had also been a feeling of warmth and safety. On this Friday night in Ontario, I longed for that sense of warmth and safety, but couldn't find purchase in my mind, no stable ground on which to plant myself. My mind began to race. I jumped to the worst-case scenario. Would this be terminal? How could it have happened to us? We were so young. I was afraid, sad, confused, and angry all at once. I wondered what would be next.

"He said it's cancer," Sara said as she began to sob. I could hear Andrew, our twenty-one-month-old son, asking his mom what was wrong as she tried to keep it together. "They want to do a radical mastectomy within the week. I can't believe this is happening to us. What did we do to deserve this? Why me? Why us?" she said, echoing my thoughts.

We were just getting started in our young adult lives. We had married in 1975, but had taken time to enjoy ourselves for a few years before deciding to have a child. Sara worked as a therapist and I worked in sports. We were settling into our careers. And then we had Andrew, who was born in 1981.

I began to feel numb as Sara went through a few more details. I told her I would catch the first flight home the next morning. I said I loved her, that we would beat this thing. And then I hung up. But my mind kept racing.

Sleep eluded me. I thought of all the years Sara and I had been together, how we had sought and already enjoyed so many adventures in our lives. I tossed and turned, then read. I turned on the television and turned it off. Nothing seemed to help as I wrestled with the most significant trauma in my adult life.

After sleeping no more than an hour-and-a-half, I decided to get up, pack, shower, and head for home.

I'm just thirty-one. I have a two-year-old son, and I spend nearly a third of the year on the road for work. What if Sara dies?

I had no family, no support systems in Denver. There was no one to lean on to help me manage. And I didn't make enough money to get the services that could help me. How could I ever manage?

That feeling of numbness came over me again and my mind was running nonstop. I checked in at the United counter and went through immigration and customs. It was surreal, as if I were on the sidelines, watching myself go through the process. I found my way to the sterile, glass-enclosed waiting area set aside for international travelers and sat down. I not only felt alone, I felt helpless. I was 1500 miles from Sara, who I knew had to be struggling with her emotions, and it would be several hours before I could get home.

The plane landed in Denver and I hurried home.

We hugged, cried, and just held each other, not just for a brief time, but for most of that Saturday. Too young to understand the situation, Andrew was nonetheless curious about the emotions he saw from his mom and dad. He knew something wasn't right and, at times, would climb up on our laps, offering his hugs and love as he sucked his thumb and held his light green blankie.

"We won't let this ruin our lives," Sara said several times. It was not so much a declaration as an attempt to convince us. "And we won't let it run our lives, either. I'll do what I have to fight it but I will not let cancer control our lives."

She was always exceptionally resilient, exhibiting an inner strength that, in part, came from being the fourth of five children who grew up on a farm. And while she appreciated nature and the farm life, she never would have wanted to live it as an adult. She loved the bustle of the city, the chance to embrace the diversity of urban living. Music, art, antiques, museums, shopping, and city zoos always held her interest far more than the simple existence of life on the farm. Sara's pronouncement that cancer would not take over our lives was also an affirmation that she planned to keep that active, vital life she loved.

The cancer industry tends to take these matters pretty seriously, and Sara's surgery, a radical mastectomy of the right breast, was scheduled immediately for the following Wednesday. I went with her to the pre-op meeting on Monday and we headed to the hospital early Wednesday morning. As morning became afternoon, she was coming around in recovery.

"He said it went well," I told her as the anesthesia cobwebs in her mind began to diminish. "We'll be okay. Just rest so we can get you home."

The uncertainty of life was slowly sinking in. Like most people, we thought we could pretty much manage our lives. Over the first eight years of our marriage, we had grown used to thinking we were in control. Suddenly we realized that we were not as much in control of our lives as we had thought.

The breast cancer epidemic was just beginning in 1983. It was unusual for a thirty-year-old woman with no personal or family history to get the disease. Sara was in good health. Other than smoking some through college, she had no factors in her life that should have increased her risk of getting cancer of any kind. Our son, Andrew, was born after a fairly routine pregnancy. Sara had breast-fed, another thing that supposedly minimized the chance of getting the disease. But cancer is a mysterious, insidious intruder, and it was invading our lives in a way that was both disquieting and confusing.

Following the mastectomy, we mulled our options. The surgery included a sampling of lymph nodes in the area adjacent to the right side of her chest. No cancer was evident in any of the nodules. The doctors, while ultimately leaving the decision to us, were quite confident in saying they felt no further treatment was needed. Radiation, chemo, and more surgery were all options. The only easy part was second-guessing. The research we reviewed had shown no real advantage to more treatment. After thoughtful consideration, we decided that we would forego any further therapy. We would closely monitor the area and, if anything out of the ordinary surfaced, we would deal with it.

The no-further-treatment approach also allowed us to hold options in reserve, in the event the cancer returned. You can only have so much radiation. And a body can stand only so much chemotherapy. Once you exhaust those options, there is little in reserve. Part of our strategy took that into account, too, as we rationalized our decision.

We thought about Sara's cancer experience from a variety of perspectives. Would it be beneficial for Sara to change her food choices? Was there some environmental influence responsible for the development of her cancer? If we thought so, should we pursue finding what could be the source? Should she have reconstruction? Were there stressors in her life that were making her more susceptible to the disease? These were questions both Sara and I wrestled with.

Much of our ability to deal with Sara's cancer was rooted in our commonsense, Midwestern upbringing.

Wauseon was a great place to grow up and things were pretty good for both of us. Neither Sara nor I came from more than a middle-class background. Her dad farmed eighty acres east of the town of about 5,000 people. Her mother was an English teacher at the local high school and, in fact, taught us English during our freshman year.

My father worked in management for a dairy that expanded to include several dozen convenience stores throughout the area surrounding and including Toledo. My mom was a housewife, cut from the cloth of June Cleaver on the *Leave It to Beaver* show.

The oldest of five children, I had three brothers and one sister. Sara's family was the reverse: four girls and a boy. Her position as fourth in the order equipped her with a wonderful personality, one of great tolerance and easygoing acceptance.

Sara attended a rural school through eighth grade and was a good student, but her greatest strength always was her ability to connect with people. She thrived on the social aspects of whatever she did, and it was reflected in a variety of extra-curricular activities in high school.

My childhood was a mosaic of school, sports, and working. I loved baseball, football, and basketball and played endlessly with friends in neighborhood backyards, parks, and driveways. From early on, I was fascinated by the administrative part of it. Figuring out how to put on the events was as much fun as playing the games. As it turned out, it was a precursor to my life's work in the world of professional sports.

After that first date during our freshman year of high school, we had gone our separate ways. We each had a close circle of friends, took our studies reasonably seriously, and enjoyed variety when it came to both experiences and friend-ships. Sara didn't date as much as I did, but by our junior year, we both decided we'd had enough of that and began to date each other on a constant basis. We were going steady for most of our final year in high school.

After high school, Sara went to Colorado State University her first year and I went to the University of Toledo.

Sara's penchant for the arts and drama led her to believe she wanted a degree in fashion merchandising. She always had a flair for knowing what went well with what and her decorat-ing skills were better than most. CSU offered a degree program in that area and she began her studies in that discipline in the fall of 1970.

I always saw myself as a writer, one with a passion for what was right, interested in helping the underdog. Investigative journalism was starting to blossom and becoming a reporter topped my list of vocational priorities, so I selected a major in journalism.

In 1970, Colorado was *the* place to be. Everyone in the Woodstock generation had visions of picking up and moving to the heart of the Rockies. Sara's first year at CSU was as much about social and cultural activities as it was academics.

For me, even though the University of Toledo was just thirty-five miles from my folks' house, that thirty-five miles meant freedom.

Being free to do as you please is one of the great joys of college life. It also is one of the great dilemmas of young adulthood. Both Sara and I wrestled with properly managing our new-found independence. Sara was a frequent visitor to her classes with mixed results in her freshman year. My first term, I checked out the opening day of classes in both Psych and Soc 101 to get the course syllabus. I read what little I could find time for in both textbooks, went to mid-terms and finals, and ended up with a D in each class. I had passed, which was okay in the pass-fail world of the early seventies.

As the end of spring rolled around, Sara and I each received an A socially, but we were both on the edge academically. We returned to Wauseon for the summer and were faced with some real soul-searching. We needed to get some focus in our lives. Neither of us was overjoyed with the relationships we had forged with the opposite sex while away. They didn't have the depth and caring we had with one another. While we did not yet want to get married, we knew we wanted to spend our college days together.

We also knew that if we were to make this college thing work, we had to abandon our current approach to academics. With grade point averages hovering around 2.0, we had come to the realization we must focus on our studies or we were wasting our time.

We were excited to be together for the summer but Sara's mother had her reservations about our relationship. Being together took on a clandestine tone. Sara would generally leave home to meet me so her mother wouldn't know we were getting together. Our favorite spot became York School, Sara's elementary and junior high school.

By summer's end, we decided we would be together following our upcoming sophomore year. We did so, made our way through college, and moved to Pueblo, Colorado, in 1976. I had just received my master's degree in sports administration from Ohio University and accepted a job as sports information director at the University of Southern Colorado.

Sara, who supported us with a job in occupational therapy at the Ohio University Affiliated Health Center while I was in grad school, moved her focus to psychiatry and took a position at the Colorado State Hospital.

In 1980 we decided the time was right to begin chasing our dream of children. As directed by our physician, we looked to wait a minimum of six months from the August day that Sara quit taking the pill. However, in late November, she became pregnant.

The pregnancy went smoothly. It was winding down in August, but Andrew wasn't ready to join us. His due date came and went. A week later he determined it was showtime.

We had just settled into our family room to watch one of the all-time great guy movies—*Caddyshack*. It was 10:30 on a Sunday night and Sara's mother, who was visiting from Ohio to be a part of Andrew's birth, was knitting in the corner of the room. Sara had joined me on the sofa.

We weren't fifteen minutes into the film when Sara wondered aloud about what was going on. The couch cushion was getting damp under her. It didn't take long to figure out that her water had broken. We hurriedly packed up our Volkswagen Rabbit and headed to the hospital. As we drove along the freeway, I looked over at her. Concern was written all over her face, but the radiance that goes with pregnancy I had seen so many times over the preceding nine months reminded me of how much I loved her.

The ride was quiet for the first few minutes as we considered the magnitude of the moment.

"You know, this is the last time it will ever be like this—just you and me," I said.

She turned toward me, smiled, and nodded. But she was preparing herself for the task before her and it was obvious she was holding on against the periodic sharp pains she experienced.

We often recalled that moment as the years passed, happy to have had that minute on southbound I-25 to help give perspective to our lives.

We enjoyed our time in Pueblo. The city was friendly, offered trouble free living, and was very affordable. But its relatively small size and lack of sophistication was growing stale, and we began to explore options elsewhere. I had considered going to law school but ended up accepting a job in public relations with the Sports Car Club of America in suburban Denver.

The Mile High City offered us the excitement of a bigger place and we had always been fans of the city a hundred miles to the north.

Andrew was twenty-one months old when Sara experienced her initial cancer episode, and I'm convinced it was instrumental in his development. It made him a person who cares deeply about others, particularly those who face challenges or are disadvantaged. But with Sara's cancer, I found that one of my biggest concerns was parenting my young son.

It was always tempting to second-guess our decisions about Sara's health. Could the doctor, who made her first cancer diagnosis, have found it sooner? Should they have been more aggressive in treating it? Would it have made a difference? Should he have insisted on additional treatment after the mastectomy? Why Sara? What was the cause? Was it genetic or something in the environment? The questions were endless.

You can make yourself crazy thinking about it. Both Sara and I had moments when we pondered our plight. But it served no real benefit. I quickly learned to put my anger, doubts, and sadness behind me. I had accepted our path and understood that, if I focused on anything less, we could easily miss so much that life has to offer.

Cancer causes a person to become a prisoner in their own body and, fortunately, it's not something many of us experience.

We can be thankful for that. But cancer puts you in that position. You're stuck. There truly are no alternatives.

Sara was always a woman of action. She did not enjoy having to sit around, waiting for test results, doctors' opinions, and other things to happen.

There's no doubt that cancer changed that for her. But Sara fought with a will that was often amazing to witness.

After her initial episode with the diagnosis and subsequent surgery, things calmed down for a bit. We discussed the possibility of reconstructive surgery. Sara's body was curvy and her breasts were a significant part of her look. She was very self-conscious about the loss of her right breast. Our culture and society places such significance on a woman's chest. Sara understood that intimately, even though I told her (and meant it) that it didn't matter to me.

"What's important is that you are here," I always said in response when she raised the reconstruction question. "It's only flesh." I didn't believe the risks and pain associated with doing it were worth it. And in 1983, the options, procedures, and technical expertise were not anywhere near what they are today.

We were ready for our lives to settle down so we could continue with our adventures. I stayed at the Sports Car Club of America for two years before taking a job heading up Motorsports Public Relations for Coors in Golden, Colorado. Sara continued her career in occupational therapy, working with adolescents at Bethesda Psychiatric Hospital.

The sports work was taxing and long hours were the rule. And unending travel was a necessary component of the job. When I was home, we spent as much time as possible with Andrew and were constantly looking to entertain him. Ironically, one of the things he seemed to enjoy most was going to Denver's Stapleton Airport to watch the many airliners come and go.

While Sara's life was busy with the fairly normal and routine, I was running around North America, attending race events and doing PR and promotional activities that accompanied them.

One of the biggest challenges with doing sports, entertainment, and event marketing is that there is little, if any, break. I was in the office on Monday, preparing for the next race. On Tuesday or Wednesday, I was off to the city where the event would take place. I generally stayed through the conclusion of the event, which was most often on a Sunday. Then it was back to the airport that night or early Monday morning. I returned to the office that afternoon, and it all started again.

In the end, I was missing much of the early, formative years in Andrew's life. And while we didn't speak of it often, Sara's cancer was bubbling beneath it all. Maybe it was good we spent so much time apart and were so busy. It undoubtedly helped minimize the concerns and doubts that remained in our minds.

Being diagnosed with cancer at thirty is by no means a death knell. But in those moments when we were brutally honest with ourselves, we knew the long-term odds were against us. There was always the unspoken question of how long we would go before the disease would again rear its ugly head. The "dandelions" were a very real part of our lives. Not many days passed when it didn't pop into my head, at least for a few moments. And it was a constant for Sara, as well. As we looked ahead, we figured cancer was something we would see again. It was a never-ending stress, always gnawing at us. Always.

One of the most interesting things was that we rarely talked about it. As much as we communicated, as connected as our lives were, we just didn't discuss it. Should it have been more a part of the conversation? Maybe. But the uncertainty associated with the unknown can be a powerful thing and we felt dwelling on it was a waste of time. We never consciously made the decision to not discuss cancer. It was an intuitive decision and one that made our day-to-day existence easier to deal with. Besides, we were busy living our lives.

As Sara had said, we couldn't let cancer run our lives. And we weren't going to let it ruin our lives.

It reminded me of those moments as a kid when your worst fear was the bogeyman lurking in the closet or the creepy monster under the bed. It was a life tinged with unease and apprehension.

It *might* seem that we could forget about it. But, then a first-time pain cropped up. An unexplainable headache surfaced or a bout with the flu came out of nowhere. Each created a concern, even as we tried to remain positive and focused on the routine of our lives.

That, coupled with my work routine, had worn me down. I had spent thirty-two weekends on the road in my first year at Coors. It was a brutal reality and there was no relief on the horizon.

Enter a colleague and friend I had worked with both at the SCCA and Coors, a young, brash IndyCar team owner named Rick Galles who had big dreams, in addition to winning races and championships. He called me as the 1985 racing season was concluding and asked me if I would be interested in working with him on another project.

"Remember how I've talked about starting a sports marketing agency?" he said, enthusiasm bubbling up in his voice. "Well, it's time."

After thinking it over and thoroughly discussing it with Sara, we decided to pursue it.

"Well, we've always said our life is an adventure," she said. "And this would be the next chapter in our journey. I think New Mexico could be a great place to live and I doubt that I will have much trouble finding a job.

While I was excited about the opportunity, I had real questions about the viability of such an effort. How would we grow it? Who would join me to staff up the organization? Would we truly be able to secure clients? Would I be left alone to run the company, as promised? How committed was Rick to this venture? The questions wouldn't go away and bounced around my head long after I accepted the job.

My discomfort ended up being well-founded. Ramping up a new company is a huge chore, and I was innocent and naïve in many ways. We slowly grew from our humble beginnings. After nine months, we were close to breaking even and things looked bright for the business. But my doubts about being second-guessed were real and growing.

What was comfortable was our family situation. Andrew was five and in preschool. Sara had little trouble locating a job, landing one with the Albuquerque Public Schools. Being the good Lutheran she was, Sara located a church and attended regularly. One of the highlights when we went was the presence of a well-to-do ranch family that had a dozen or so kids, almost all Korean. Sara got to know the mother of the clan and learned they had adopted the children after their naturally born children had become adults.

Sara found the Korean kids adorable and began working on me to consider adoption. I was somewhat ambivalent about it, being content with Andrew. Having a second child was not a priority for me. But Sara felt differently.

If we did want to add to our family, adoption had become our only option. Sara was constantly learning about the many effects of breast cancer. It was not a good idea for her estrogen to be elevated. Pregnancy elevated estrogen. Having another child was not a good idea. Once we arrived at and accepted that conclusion, the decision came pretty easily. I told her I would get a vasectomy and then she could discontinue using birth control pills—another concern due to the estrogen in the compound.

A few days passed and she and I talked one night after we had put Andrew to bed.

"I have been thinking about you having a vasectomy and I think I have a better option," Sara said. "I should do sterilization. That way, if my cancer recurs and something happens to me, you can marry again and will be able to have kids with your new wife."

It was so like her. Sara was always thinking of others.

"No, I'll do the vasectomy," I countered. "It's a simple procedure and I'll be back to normal in no time."

But she would not relent.

"No," she said firmly, "you need the option available to you if you ever get remarried and your wife wants kids. It's clear to me that sterilization is the way to go. I have accepted that I won't have any more children and I'm okay with it."

She was right. If she died and I got remarried, it would be best to have the option.

The next day, she arranged the procedure and, within the month, it was done. It was a thoughtful and prudent approach. But it was also another reminder of her ongoing bout with cancer.

It was always there, nibbling at our psyches. We tried to push cancer to the deepest recesses of our minds, and often could. But cancer's tentacles had snaked their way into our lives, and they would never let go.

The Five Star business was going okay, but I had grown weary of being micromanaged.

I talked with Sara and we decided it was time for me to quietly start looking to make a move. Neither of us saw the experience as a failure, nor did we have any regrets. We saw it as yet another chapter in our adventures.

As I worked my network, I discovered an option existed back in Denver. We could return, move back into our Littleton home, and regain the traction we had lost when we moved to Albuquerque.

I returned to the Sports Car Club of America as director of marketing in January of 1987. Sara quickly landed an OT job with Denver Public Schools.

It was good to be back in Denver. The Mile High City truly felt like home. It harbored tough memories from Sara's initial bout with cancer, but it also served as a solid foundation for the next chapter in our journey.

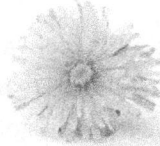

CHAPTER
3

While moving monopolized our attention, Sara had not retreated from her interest in adoption. She had studied agencies, procedures, and processes and discovered what she believed to be the right group in Denver. It was an organization called Friends of Children of Various Nations (FCVN) and was located just a few blocks east of downtown.

In early June, she came to me one day after work and raised the adoption question once more. I was extremely busy with my new job and really had not given much thought to the question.

But Sara had.

She asked me if I had thought more about it and if I was still okay with it. I told her I was. She talked about FCVN and added that we would have to participate in FCVN's orientation if we were to adopt.

"Sounds good to me," I offered, mulling all the work I had going as I half listened to her rambling through the information about the process. "Just let me know when you think we might want to start the process."

As usual, she had already done so.

"I already signed us up for the next orientation," she said, her eyes twinkling as they did when she was running with a plan. Now she had my attention.

"You did, huh?" I said with a smile. "Don't you think you could have asked me first?"

"You're always so busy. If I'd asked, you would have tried to put it off," she replied, giving me a playful poke in the ribs. "I knew you were on board with it and, if we were ever going to get going with this, it was up to me to make it happen."

I could have objected but knew it was fruitless. She had her heart set on making this a reality. I knew it was time to get my head in the adoption game. This was just sooner than I had expected.

"When does it start?" I asked with resignation.

"We have to go July 4th weekend," she said. "I have arranged for Andrew to stay with friends on those days. It sounds like it's pretty intense for a couple of days."

"I guess it's good to know they are screening people in a serious way," I said. "God knows there are a lot of people with kids who don't know how to parent very well."

Sara looked at me with a gleam in her brown eyes. She said that based on her research, she thought we would be able to request, and get, a little girl since we already had a son. She added that most kids being adopted through FCVN were from Korea.

"I always think about those kids in our church in Albuquerque and how cute they all were," she continued. "We'll get a little girl just like one of those."

I couldn't do anything but pull her close and hug her.

"You're right," I said. "We'll be getting a little girl that will be so cute. I'm sorry if I seem distracted and sort of distant about all this."

July 4th weekend we went for our orientation. FCVN was housed in a converted Victorian home on the west edge of City Park and not far from the city's hospital district.

The process of adoption was far more involved than we had expected. It was comforting to know the agency was committed to extensive background checks and comprehensive sessions to determine if a couple's parenting skills were appropriate for adoption.

As our sessions played out, it became obvious there was a diversity of parenting capabilities in the group. In the end, two couples were deemed to not be candidates for adoption. Following the session in which the first couple had been eliminated, Sara and I climbed into the car and were quiet as we headed to our suburban home. I broke the silence as we entered the freeway.

"I can't imagine what it would be like to go through all they have as part of this and then be told the agency has decided you aren't a good candidate to be a parent. It would be terrible."

As the next few weeks passed, we received our approval and in late 1987, we were placed in line for a child. Sara and I were firm in our request for a Korean girl. We also said we would be willing to take a special needs child, as long as the condition was medically correctible.

In early February, we received a letter saying the agency had identified a baby girl that was at an agency in Seoul. She was born January 8 and in a foster home due to a heart condition. If we were interested in learning more, we were to contact the agency and would get a picture and more information.

"I don't want us to get ahead of ourselves, but I have a good feeling about this," Sara said. "I will get in touch with the agency first thing in the morning and see what we can find out."

Late the following morning, I returned to my office from a meeting to find a note to call Sara. I quickly rang her up and she answered, excitement in her voice.

"I went to FCVN and picked up the photo and a little more information," she said, enthusiasm oozing from her voice. "Ron, she is so cute. You won't believe it. I can't wait to show you her picture."

I went through the rest of my work day often thinking of the call and left the office earlier than normal so I could be with her. I walked into the kitchen to find Sara sorting through papers and looking at the photo.

"Look. Isn't she beautiful?" she said, smiling with tears coming to her eyes. "I can't believe how gorgeous she is."

I held the picture and studied it. Her round face was kind of cute, I thought. Black hair was sticking out in a dozen directions and her eyes were nearly closed. Well, she was a baby, I thought. Cute, but beautiful? I didn't know about that.

"She's very cute," I finally said, deferring to Sara's enthusiasm.

"I can see it in her features and face. She'll be a beautiful girl and woman," Sara gushed.

My focus turned to the paperwork and the limited background we had. Her name was Park Keyong-Og. Park was her last name. Keyong-Og, we were told in the background information, meant "shiny glass bead."

"I'm curious about her heart condition," I said. "What does it say here and what else did you find out?"

"They have diagnosed it as an atrial septal defect, a hole in the wall between the lower chambers of her heart. I already talked to our doctor about it, and he said it should be something that is correctible. He will refer us to a heart specialist at Children's Hospital after examining her. I talked to our insurance, too, and they'll cover it."

It was obvious that Sara had already decided. It all sounded good, but this was a big decision. Andrew, who had a pretty big stake in this, had been watching and listening to us talk. It was time to get his six-year-old opinion.

"So what do you think, Scooze?" I said to him.

"She looks like she's nice, Dad," he said.

"Do you think you'd like to have her as a sister?"

"I think so," he said in a way that told me he was ready to move onto something else. He then brought us all back to reality.

"Mom, I'm hungry. When are we going to eat?"

Sara and I looked at each other and laughed. Life may change—even change dramatically—but there's always a question to answer, a meal to make.

"Let's think about this tonight and make a decision tomorrow," I said. "But I think I know where this is going to end up," I added with a laugh.

The next few months were a whirlwind as we prepared to welcome a daughter to our family. Sara and I often laughed about how this was absolutely *the* way to have a child, *especially* from the mom's perspective.

We prepared the bedroom and began to gather girlie clothes. We talked about names and narrowed it to a couple. It would be Emily—which is what Andrew would have been had he been a girl—or Jenny, short for Jennifer. We decided on Jenny.

We also spent a lot of time talking with Andrew about his new sister. His easygoing demeanor made the process less difficult. From early on, he had been thoughtful and discerning. He also was very attentive and often asked questions that seemed far beyond his years.

The agency kept us informed of Keyong-Og's status. Her overall health was okay but the heart condition was preventing her from gaining weight as she should. The agency assured us the paperwork was in process to get her into the US and to finalize the adoption.

The timeline for us to get her to Denver was coming together and we figured the end of May was a realistic goal. FCVN told us that a group of flight attendants regularly worked with adoption agencies to bring children to the US. We appreciated having the option but we ultimately decided to go to Seoul to pick her up.

This was one time I was happy I had spent all that time on the road. I had amassed a huge number of United Airlines Premier miles and a fraction of them could be transformed into first-class tickets. We secured our passports and prepped for our long trip. A couple days before we left, FCVN asked us to come by the office so we could take a duffle bag filled with supplies it had gathered for its Korean counterpart.

We arranged for Andrew to stay with friends during our time in the Far East.

"We're going to miss you," said Sara as we tucked him into his bed the night before we left. His bedroom was like those of many six-year-old boys in 1988. A poster of Mr. T was on the back of his door. Numerous He-Man characters populated his room. A Denver Broncos poster was on the wall and a soccer ball and mini-basketball hoop were in one corner.

"I'll miss you guys, too," he said, tears coming to his eyes.

"Hey Scooze, you'll have a great time with your buddy Eric and his family," I said. "And when we come back, you'll come to the airport and meet your new sister."

A thoughtful look came across his face. "Do you think she will want to eat just rice? Will she know karate and how to use Ninja swords?"

Sara and I looked at each other and couldn't help but laugh. Andrew had brought this up previously when we discussed the adoption and his sister coming from Korea.

"Where do you get these ideas?" Sara said, knowing the answer.

"I saw it in a movie," he said, a little embarrassed after Sara and I had laughed at his comment. "Everybody there knows kung fu and karate. And they do eat lots of rice, right?"

The power of media and the stereotypical suggestions it engenders, I thought.

"I doubt she will have swords or nunchucks," I said with a smile as I tousled his red hair.

"Good night, Mom. Good night, Dad. I love you." We left him to sleep and continued to discuss the transition he faced.

"He's going to be fine," I said. "It's just a lot for him to digest right now."

"Another chapter for us," Sara reminded me as we reached our bedroom. "It seems like a long time ago when I first saw all those Korean kids in Albuquerque. Look where it led us."

We got up early Monday morning and headed to Denver's Stapleton Airport.

After two flights and a long day of travel, we arrived in Seoul on Tuesday afternoon. Like many Asian cities, Seoul is a massive place. The South Korean capital was in the final stages of preparing for the 1988 Summer Olympics, and the national pride of such a small country, as it prepared for its place on the world stage, was omnipresent. Thousands of banners, billboards, and street signs lined the route from Kimpo Airport to the hotel. We were worn out by all the travel, and jet lag made it difficult to get as much sleep as we needed. We awoke early Wednesday and got ready for our first meeting with our baby daughter. We arrived at the agency carrying the massive green duffle bag we had toted along.

The agency director came into the lobby and greeted us, smiling and speaking very broken English. She told us that the agency was bringing Keyong-Og and her foster mother to meet us and they should arrive shortly. We waited nervously in a conference room. Shortly after we sat down, one of the staff returned, holding a heavily blanketed baby.

Sara stood and moved toward her. The young woman smiled and handed Keyong-Og to her. Sara inched the blankets back from her face. She was asleep and didn't stir.

I moved to Sara's side and she turned to me, tears streaming down her cheeks.

"She's every bit as beautiful as I thought she would be," she said. "I can't believe we actually are here and I'm holding her."

I stayed in the background and let Sara have her moment. She held Jenny for another minute before turning to me and handing her over. I took her in my arms and looked into her face. She remained asleep, largely a function, I suspected, of the heart condition that had kept her five-month-old weight at an anemic eight pounds.

Our agency contact told us that we could talk with the doctor who had examined Jenny initially and diagnosed her condition. We passed Jenny back and forth for the next half hour before the young woman said the foster mother and Keyong-Og needed to return to her home.

We went to an adjacent office where we met with the doctor, who spoke very basic English. It was obvious, though, that she was fully confident in her diagnosis. Sara and I thanked her and left. The young woman from the agency escorted us to the lobby.

"I wanted to take her with us right now," said Sara. "I still am trying to process all this. We have a daughter! Can you believe it?"

I was trying to get my head around it all, as well.

"I feel the same," I said. "It seems like we should have her now. But we'll all be together soon. And, the good thing is, in the interim, we can spend time being tourists in the country where she was born. We can see and do things that we will tell her about later."

Our second encounter with Jenny came Saturday.

The streets were very busy and the driver fought his way through the chaotic thoroughfares. We sat in the van and soaked in the seemingly endless, incredible energy of this magnificent city. It was a warm and sunny late May day and the van's windows were open. The sounds of traffic, the bustling pedestrians, and the smell of kimchi surrounded us. The driver wound his way into a residential neighborhood that sat behind rows of shops. He drove as far as he could before stopping and turning to our guide. He spoke to her in Korean and when he finished, she turned to us and said, "We have a short walk to her home."

We followed the young woman up a winding walkway that led to the front door of a house built into the hillside. The middle-aged woman we had seen at the agency opened the door, ushered us in, and led us across beautiful hardwood floors to a room in the middle of her house. Jenny was wrapped in three blankets, sleeping comfortably on a mat, centered on the floor. Sara's first instinct was to pick her up, but she waited.

The foster mother and our escort conversed for a few moments and the foster mom picked Jenny up. She turned to Sara and, in a moment only mothers can understand, handed Jenny to her.

Sara's first movement was to pull the blankets back from Jenny's face. She rustled, but didn't awaken. Her dark black hair was matted with perspiration. Sara held her closely and I could see her eyes starting to tear. After holding her for what seemed like several minutes, she offered her to me and I cradled her in my arms. She seemed so small, so slight for her age. The heart condition was doing its best to keep her from growing.

We enjoyed our brief visit and were pleased we had the memory to eventually share with Jenny. We thanked the foster mother several times as we left. We finalized our plans to pick up Jenny on Monday.

Our departure day arrived and we were excited to be at the agency to pick up Jenny and begin our long journey back to Colorado.

The director and the female guide were there to greet us. We sat for a few minutes before the foster mother appeared with Jenny in her arms. She smiled but the moisture that was in her eyes served as an indicator that this was not easy for her. We again thanked the foster mother for all she had done. She kissed Keyong-Og on the forehead and said good-bye.

When we left and were headed to the airport, Sara removed the layers of blankets from Jenny. She was in a footed sleeper and her little face was beaded with sweat.

"I know they were doing what they felt is best for her," Sara said, "but this bundling her has to stop. She is constantly sweating; she has to be uncomfortable."

We arrived at the airport and went through immigration and customs. Jenny's red South Korean passport was the ticket to her new life half a world away. About ten hours later, we landed in Seattle, cleared immigration and customs, and headed off to our Denver flight. We still had nearly two-and-a-half hours to Denver, but it felt good to be back in the US.

Jenny had been pretty quiet throughout. We discovered over the next several days that she had learned to pace herself, and that meant sleeping for much of the day. She used a significant amount of energy to process her formula. I quickly found that when feeding her a bottle, the sleeve of my long-sleeved shirt would be soaked with her sweat from wrist to bicep, where her head rested. Her body was struggling to get blood to her stomach to aid in the digestion process.

As we began our descent into Denver, our thoughts turned to Andrew. We had talked several times over the past week about how he was doing and wondered how he would adapt to having a new sister. We had phoned once to talk briefly with him and he seemed fine.

Sara and I had gone through a life-altering experience the past week. His was about to start.

Unlike me, Sara looked terrific as the plane hit the runway. Holding Jenny, she appeared absolutely radiant—that new mom look. We rolled toward the gate and were the first people off the plane. We walked up the jetway and emerged to see Andrew running toward us. He yelled out, "Mom, Dad," and jumped into my arms. Even though he was six years old, he wasn't too old—yet—to show his affection in public.

"Do you want to see your new sister?" asked Sara.

Andrew dropped from my hug to stand and look into his mom's arms. His face was stoic as he examined the newest member of the Richards family.

"She's so little," he said. "She's dinky." It was a nickname he used for her through the first several years of her life.

Jenny was unfazed by it all, sleeping soundly as her new brother studied her. We kneeled and did a group hug as our friends looked on.

Later, as darkness fell, I helped Andrew get ready for bed. Sara was in Jenny's room, checking on her as Andrew climbed into bed. He turned to me with a quizzical look. I couldn't wait to hear what he would ask.

"Do you think Jenny knows me yet?" he asked. "I don't think she knows I'm her brother."

"You know, she's just getting to know all of us," I said. "It'll take a little bit of time for that to happen, but it should pretty quickly. She's gone through lots of changes in a very short period of time. Plus, you can't forget what we said about her heart not being perfect."

He looked more deeply into my eyes and answered, "Yes, I know."

"It makes her very tired," I said. "We'll take her to the doctor soon and see what we need to do, but I think she'll need to have an operation."

"Will Jenny's heart be okay?" he said with genuine concern.

Sara had been standing in the doorway and moved in to sit down beside me.

"I'm sure she'll be fine," she said. Andrew seemed comforted by his mother's words and settled in to go to sleep.

"Okay, Mom," he said. "I'm glad you think so. Good night."

"He is really concerned about her," I said, as we left his room. "He asked me about her heart, too. He's going to be such a good brother."

"I've seen a lot of kids with health conditions, you know, and I think she soon could reach a stage where she begins to fail to thrive," Sara said. "We need to get her to the doctor soon."

Sara took Jenny to our family physician the next day and, after examining her, he excused himself from the exam room. He returned and said he had spoken to a pediatric cardiologist at Children's Hospital. He told her that he didn't think the situation was critical, but it was serious and he wanted Jenny to have a few more tests. He asked Sara to leave his office and head to Children's for the tests.

I met Sara at the hospital shortly thereafter. The doctors ordered an ultrasound to get an idea of the damage in her heart. It showed what had been diagnosed in Seoul, a hole in the wall separating the lower chambers. It was causing blood to swish back and forth with each heartbeat, minimizing the organ's effectiveness.

The cardiologist, one of the best surgeons in the country, was a big man—well over six feet tall, before you took the cowboy boots into account.

"There's no reason to worry, but we need to repair this sooner rather than later," he said calmly. "We'll schedule her for surgery as soon as possible and get this done so she can get on with growing and living a normal life."

A couple of weeks later, Jenny went in for the operation. The surgeon did his superb work, using a small Kevlar patch to seal the hole. He also closed a second, small hole and snipped a muscle band he found wrapped around her aorta so it wouldn't restrict her heart's function. After a few days in the ICU, and a couple more in the nursery, we brought Jenny home.

The "zipper" on her chest was testament to the significance of the surgery. She immediately began to gain weight and, while she seemed to be slightly behind in several areas of development, Sara and I were confident the heart issue was resolved.

As she gained strength, Jenny became much more active. She learned to walk at about a year, but her speech was delayed a bit longer. She would often point to something and squeal, letting us know she wanted whatever the object of her attention was.

While Jenny's health improved, it was becoming apparent that she could be a difficult child. We worked hard to create a strong bond and those efforts seemed to be working. What was puzzling was that we could do little, if anything, to soothe her. A typical situation would occur during dinner. She would get agitated about something, start to scream, throw her food dish or some food, and then start to cry. We changed her environment, held her, talked to her, and did everything we could to quiet her. Little seemed to help. It was as if she had to cry herself out, physically wearing herself down, before she would once again become quiet.

In addition to her delayed speech, we found it odd that she rarely let us read to her. She seemed to want to control the book and did not really listen. When she was older, she listened to enough of the story to get a handle on it and, when she had a grasp of it, she would take the book and "read" the story to us. We thought it odd, especially after having Andrew, who would sit quietly and soak in the stories. Not Jenny.

As she continued to grow, we realized the heart condition was not the only special need to deal with. Something even more difficult awaited us as she aged.

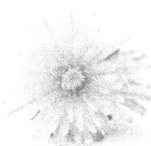

CHAPTER
4

Another move was in our future in early 1989. I was contacted about a job opportunity in Milwaukee, and it led to me accepting the position leading the Sports Marketing Public Relations function at Miller Brewing Company.

I started in March. Sara and I decided I would move ahead, leaving her and the kids in Denver so Andrew could finish out the school year.

Just a few days after starting my job, I called Sara for our nightly check-in. We traded small talk and it seemed something was bothering her. I asked if everything was all right and she hesitated but then said she had made an appointment with her doctor after discovering a small lump in her right chest area.

I swallowed hard and thought about how quickly life can change. Was her cancer back? Or was it a false alarm? We could only hope it was a benign mass. A sinking feeling of fear washed over me and settled in my stomach. I was angry that this had occurred again in our lives. I wondered why, just as I had on that day six years before in Canada. I did my best to quash my emotions. It would not help Sara as she did her best to deal with her feelings.

The timing couldn't have been much worse. Sara was working full-time and managing the kids, totally on her own. I couldn't really ask for time off to be with her, being that I was a thousand miles away and just a few days into my new job.

"I'll be okay. I've thought about it and I can manage," she said. "I'll find out what they want to do and go from there. Remember, as I have always said, cancer doesn't run our lives."

What could I do but agree with her. She was being her usually resilient and strong self and needed me to say I agreed. I did, but not without reservations. I could already feel a swelling sense of guilt for not being there with her to help.

A few days later, her surgeon removed the small mass in an out-patient procedure. We were not surprised that the biopsy confirmed it was cancerous. Our time away from the disease ended six years after it started.

Sara was matter-of-fact about it when we spoke the evening of the surgery.

"Well, now we know what we're up against," she said. "I have to say, I had a false sense of security when I reached the five-year milestone. I was clear for more time than that, and now this happens. You can never figure you are out of the woods . . ." she said, her voice trailing off.

Cancer was back in our lives and, like it or not, it was running things for the next couple of months.

After healing from the relatively minor surgery, Sara started her treatments. Her oncologist prescribed radiation and hyperthermia, a procedure in which they heat the affected area to around 110 degrees. The radiation was tolerable, although it made Sara tired. The hyperthermia was something else. The technician would attach a lead to a device implanted in her chest. Electricity warmed the device and Sara would only describe it as torture.

One evening as we talked, she went off about the whole process. It was unusual to hear her so upset.

"The technician is always talking to me, trying to distract me," she said, annoyed with the way that day's treatment had played out. "And he does it while raising the temperature. It goes way beyond being uncomfortable. It just plain hurts. I can't wait until this is over."

She managed to handle the remaining treatments. But she headed back to work with her adolescent patients at the psych hospital after every treatment, making it all the more difficult. I returned to Colorado every other weekend, and it was clear Sara needed the break. She was worn to a frazzle. Working, caring for the kids, and getting ready to move were a ton to deal with. Throw in the mental strain of another round with cancer and the treatments, and Sara was hanging by a thread.

She somehow got through the entire episode. She and the kids joined me in Wisconsin in June. We were in a temporary living apartment for a couple of weeks. Having two kids and a cat in less than nine hundred square feet after being in a house for the past ten years was a real challenge.

Unfortunately, the real estate market in Denver was such that it made no sense for us to attempt to sell our home. Its value was thirty percent less than we had paid for it just a few years earlier. Compounding the problem was that I was coming to Miller at a level that did not allow them to purchase our home. We decided to rent it for a time, hoping the Denver market would rebound.

We looked in earnest for a rental house in a very tight market and finally moved into a home in Thiensville, a quaint suburb north of Milwaukee. It was a very old home, very different from what we were used to. As we had done when we moved to Albuquerque, we were compromising on our home choice. It was a frustration that lingered for several years.

One day in late summer of 1989, I slipped away from the office early and headed home. Sara was at work and the kids were at daycare, so it was quiet around the big, old house. I got the mail and sat down at the kitchen table to look through it while having a Miller Lite. In the middle of the stack of envelopes was one from a bank card that I didn't recognize. It was addressed to Sara and I was curious since it was an account I had not seen before. My curiosity got the best of me and I opened the envelope. It was a bill with a balance of nearly $4,000, and the detail in the statement indicated it was for charges for a doctor's services.

When Sara arrived that evening, we went about our parental duties. After we had eaten, Sara gathered the trash and took it to the garage. I followed her out to the trash bins, taking the credit card bill with me. She turned after stuffing the plastic bag in the bin and was startled to find me walking toward her. She asked if everything was okay.

"I wanted to ask you about this," I said, more curious than anything else as I held up the bill in my right hand.

"What is it?" she said.

"That's what I'm wondering. I found it as I went through the mail today," I said, trying not to sound accusatory. "It's a credit card bill for almost $4,000. I wondered because it's an account I haven't seen before."

Sara was obviously uncomfortable as she looked at the invoice. When she looked at me, tears were forming in her eyes.

"It's an account I opened. I didn't want you to know about it."

Now I was very curious. "Why didn't you want me to know about it?"

"Because it shows the cost of my appointments with a psychologist," she said. "I started in Denver and I have continued to see someone here. I didn't want you to know because I don't want you to think I can't handle everything."

She was seeing a doctor off our insurance and had opened an account to pay for it so I wouldn't know. I was confused but mostly sensed the pain she must have been feeling as she tried, on her own, to manage all on her plate. I moved toward her and hugged her as she began to cry.

"With everything I had going on in Denver—trying to keep up with the kids, working, doing my treatments, keeping up the house, missing you—it all became too much for me. You are so busy with work. You didn't need to be worried that I couldn't manage it all."

I felt terrible. She had been hiding this from me because she didn't want to bother me.

"You know that we always talk about things, that we work through things together," I said, trying not to sound like a parent scolding her. "I can't help, though, if I don't know about it. You and the kids are the most important thing in the world to me and anything I do, work-wise, is done to better provide for the family. You know that.

"I know," she said, resignation in her voice. "And being here in Milwaukee will be great for us, I know. But all of it, coupled with my cancer coming back, became just too much to handle. I hope you understand."

"It's understandable that you feel this way," I said, reaching out to hug her, "but I am disappointed you didn't talk with me about it."

"I know. It never works when we are less than open with each other," she said as she hugged me more tightly. "I'm relieved that you know. I hate it when we have secrets. I should have said something, I know, but I don't want you to think I'm losing it."

We walked back toward the house, our arms wrapped around one another. Hearing Jenny's loud voice brought us back to the reality of our duties as a mom and dad.

"You know the greatest thing about having the relationship we have?" I asked. "It's being there for one another. We always have been and always will be. This isn't a problem, but let's not hide things from each other, okay?"

"Agreed," Sara said, as she wiped her eyes. "We better get inside and see what Jenny's up to."

We walked up the steps, hand-in-hand, and resumed tending to the kids.

Cancer had struck again. We had effectively pushed it to the backs of our minds over the past several years. We had stuffed it away, much like sticking an old jacket in the back of the closet, next to that pair of skis last used ten years ago and you couldn't bring yourself to give away. Unlike those things, though, cancer had a way of pushing its way to the forefront and forcing its presence back into our lives.

Cancer may have reinserted its presence in our lives but, fortunately, the Tamoxifin prescribed by Sara's oncologist was working as expected. The imminent cancer threat was diminished and we felt we could, once more, move on with our lives. Sara had landed a good OT job and the world slipped back into a routine.

The kids were settling in, too. Andrew was making lots of friends and was very involved in sports, as well as his academics. Jenny was doing all right, too, and we were happy that life appeared to be going along without many bumps.

Jenny was every bit as cute as Sara suspected and people continually noticed her. One very memorable moment came when she was two years old and the four of us had gone to an event in Milwaukee. We were at the Bradley Center, a 20,000-seat arena, and the crowd was milling about, heading to their seats.

We were picking our way through the crowd and I decided a more expedient way to get through the throng was to put Jenny on my shoulders. We had walked maybe twenty yards when I felt her being pulled backwards. I quickly stopped, whirled around, and found a middle-aged woman holding Jenny's arm, pulling at her in a tug of war kind of way.

"What are you doing?" I said in a loud voice that conveyed my surprise and building anger. Sara joined me, Andrew at hand.

"Oh, I didn't mean anything by it," the woman said. "She is just so cute, like a little Oriental doll! I just had to touch her. I'm sorry"

I was stunned. Jenny was cute, deserving of some attention. But to almost be pulled from my grasp? Had this woman ever learned about personal space? And what would she have done with Jenny had she pulled her from my shoulders?

Jenny's hold on people grew as she got older. When she was four, we were on our way to visit family in Ohio and stopped at an outlet mall along the way. We were browsing through a store's clothing section when Jenny began running wildly through the store, out of control, touching all the racks of clothing. Sara and I were trying to corral her and settle her down when a young store clerk came to the section where Jenny was running and said, "She's okay. She's so cute and just precious. She can't hurt anything."

Sara and I looked at one another, then at Jenny, who had momentarily stopped. Jenny smiled an almost evil smile and then began running again. It was as if she were taunting us. And she was getting validation from a stranger. We finally rounded her up and took her to the car.

Sara was strapping her into her car seat and Jenny was still racing. She kicked at Sara and tried to hit her.

"We need to get going," I said. Andrew had trailed behind us and climbed into the minivan.

"I'll sit back here with her," Sara said, nodding her head and looking to me for support.

Andrew was ten and, as usual, was quietly getting into his seat and belting himself in.

Jenny finally quieted down several miles down the road. Sara and I talked about it later as Jenny slept soundly in her car seat. We wondered what we could do when she got like that. There didn't seem to be any way of controlling her. It was as if she fed off her own energy to get even more wound up.

Over the next couple of years, we watched as Jenny cycled up and down. She was okay for seven or eight months and then had a major meltdown.

Unfortunately, the intensity of her episodes seemed to be increasing as she aged.

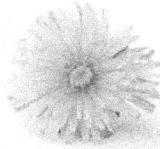

CHAPTER

5

While Jenny seemed to be spiraling up, Sara's cancer appeared to be in check. The Tamoxifan, a relatively new drug, was working. Sara's frequent blood tests and never ending exams indicated the surgery and treatments in Denver, coupled with the drug, were doing what they were designed to do. The dandelions were being held at bay.

Sara's cancer battle had declined in intensity and we were grateful. But now our worries shifted to Jenny. Her strong and sometimes defiant personality was continuing to develop, and it was becoming obvious that she had issues we needed to address. The suspicions we had about her ability to cope when she was less than a year old had spun up into full-blown concern.

By age four, Jenny had become a kid to be reckoned with at her Thiensville daycare center and she had even been termed somewhat of a bully by a couple of the children. It was not unusual to pick her up and have her start a conversation by saying, "I've got something really bad to tell you . . ." or, "You're not going to like what I have to say." Then she would describe a scenario in which she had gotten into an argument, fought with or bitten someone, or had been placed in time-out. Fortunately, the women who ran the center were very understanding and worked with us to manage Jenny and keep her on as even a keel as possible. It was no small task.

The change of scenery seemed to help some when she started kindergarten and she did relatively well until second grade. By then, her opposition to our limits and general parenting, and her often intense defiance in doing so, was becoming a problem.

It came to a head one night during the winter of 1995. Jenny had been acting out and getting in trouble at school. We'd been forced to place her in time-out on an increasing basis and were perplexed by it all. We had contacted a psychologist who specialized in childhood psychiatric disorders and were waiting to take Jenny in for an evaluation and testing.

On this particular night, we managed to get Jenny to bed around 9:00 p.m. and Andrew soon followed. Sara and I climbed into bed around 11:00 and quickly fell asleep. Around 2:00 in the morning, the door to our bedroom slowly swung open and light from the hallway flooded in on me. I awoke and saw Jenny standing in the doorway. It was a surreal scene as she stood there, backlit by the overhead light in the hall.

"Jen, are you okay?" I asked as I tried to shake the sleepiness from my head. She didn't answer. "Jenny, what's wrong?"

She didn't move from the doorway but began to speak. "I'm going to get a knife and kill you and Mom. And then I am going to kill myself," she said in a low, unnatural, almost growling voice that I had never heard from her before.

When she turned and left, I shook Sara awake and quickly told her about what I had witnessed. We jumped from bed and walked the few steps to Jenny's room. The door was cracked open and I could see she had returned to her bed. We went in and found her sleeping, breathing normally, and looking almost angelic in the same hallway light that had framed her so dramatically just a minute or so before. I began to wonder if I had imagined it all.

We sat on the edge of Jenny's bed and tried to wake her. She finally stirred, slowly opened her eyes, and asked what was wrong.

"Jenny, you just came to our room a couple of minutes ago," I said. "Do you remember that?"

She looked at me with a puzzled expression. "No, I have been here in bed, sleeping."

"Do you remember having any dreams?" I asked.

"No. Why? Did something happen?" she asked, beginning to sense she was in trouble.

"No, everything is okay. You just go back to sleep," I replied.

"We love you, Jenny," Sara said.

"I love you, too, Mom," Jenny said as she rolled away from us to go back to sleep.

Sara and I returned to our room and crawled back in bed. Sara switched on her bedside light and turned to me. I remained shaken by the incident and was now completely focused on what I had seen.

"That really had to be unbelievable," she said, now fully awake.

"It was. It reminded me of that scene with the little girl in the movie *Poltergeist*," I said. "Her voice was creepy and she sounded very determined. It was almost like she was possessed."

Sara sighed and looked away. She had shouldered much of the weight of Jenny's oppositional behavior and it was obvious it was wearing heavily on her.

"We need to get her in for an evaluation as soon as we can," she said. "She's spiraling downward, often becoming agitated for little or no reason. She's becoming more and more difficult to manage," she said, her voice trailing off.

I was still trying to process the fact that my daughter had threatened to kill her mother and me, not to mention herself. As usual, Sara was focused on the right track; we needed to get Jenny into a professional therapist as soon as possible.

Jenny continued to become more and more difficult to deal with. Her teachers were seeing it on a regular basis and contacted us on a couple of occasions.

One evening, when I returned home from work and pulled into the garage, I heard yelling and screaming coming from the house. I rushed inside and what I found was a scene that would be repeated numerous times over the next several years.

Jenny was face down on the living room floor. Sara was straddling the back of her thighs and holding her arms behind her back. Our seven-year-old was swearing at Sara, calling her names that would make a sailor blush. Tears were streaming down Sara's face as she restrained our daughter.

"She has been totally out of control, threatening me, trying to destroy things in the house, trying to hit me, bite me, kick me," Sara said.

I wasn't quite sure what to do. I wanted to help, but didn't know how.

"Where's Andrew?" I asked as Jenny called her mother a "bitch" and demanded she get off her. Jenny struggled to get away and seemingly would do anything to break free. Sara's training during years at the psychiatric hospital in Pueblo had become a necessary and welcome element of dealing with our out of control seven-year-old.

"I think he's in his room," she said, as she held tightly to Jenny's wrists.

"How long has this been going on?" I asked.

"She was very gamey—making threats and calling me names—when she got home from school. I had to restrain her about twenty minutes ago after she tried to kick and hit me."

"Are you okay?" I asked, my mind spinning from all that was happening.

"I'm all right for the moment. Go back and see how Andrew is," she suggested as Jenny continued to weakly writhe beneath her.

I walked down the hall to Andrew's room. His door was closed and he was inside, working on his homework.

"Hey Scooze," I said as I opened his door. "Are you all right?"

"Yeah, I'm okay. Is Mom okay? Jenny was just going crazy. It was scary."

It had to be frightening for him to see his sister going off as she had. I did what I could to reassure him.

"We know how Jenny can be," I said. "Mom and I are doing what is best for her. We'll get her to see a doctor and figure this out."

"I hope so," he said. "I don't like Mom sitting on her like she is. Will that hurt Jenny?"

"No," I said.

Andrew's easygoing, calm demeanor was a stark contrast to Jenny's roller-coaster personality. He had seen Jenny be extremely difficult, but his love for her never wavered.

"Mom used to work with kids who had problems like Jenny's and she knows how to control and restrain her without hurting her," I said. "Jenny isn't in any danger. But we have to help her when she can't manage herself."

It was a mantra that we would repeat many times in the coming years.

He went back to his math homework and I returned to the living room, where Sara remained atop Jenny. The intensity was quickly dissipating. Over the next few minutes, I watched as Jenny slipped completely out of her agitated state and became a frightened little girl who had no idea why she was behaving as she was. As she lay with her face against the carpet, she physically relaxed and began to cry. Sara carefully released her arms, stood, and went to the sofa. Jenny remained on the floor for another couple of minutes then rose, went to Sara, and crawled into her lap. She was sobbing as she apologized over and over again, saying she did not know why she had acted as she did.

A sense of relief settled over us for the moment. Jenny cried for several more minutes and then dozed off. The episode had drained her physically. Sara carried her into her room and got her undressed and into her pajamas. Jenny barely stirred as she did so.

We agreed that Jenny was getting worse and knew we must get her in for an evaluation. Sara felt helpless, and it scared her when she compared Jenny's behavior to that of the many kids with whom she had worked.

I shared Sara's anguish. We were scared—for Jenny and ourselves. The fact that Sara saw Jenny's behavior as similar to that of the kids she had dealt with was sobering. At the state hospital she had provided therapy for kids as young as nine who had severe mental illness. A couple of them had killed someone. I quickly did what I could to suppress the visuals that appeared in my mind. At that point, all we could do was try to manage her behavior, since she couldn't do it on her own. We believed we would figure it out, but we also knew that it was going to take some time.

By the end of the week all appeared to be good. Jenny seemed even-keeled, but Sara thought she was distant and on edge much of the time, very quiet and distracted. Jenny seemed different than she'd been even a month earlier and we felt like we were constantly walking on eggshells.

We went to bed and had been asleep about three hours when we heard Jenny yelling and crying. Sara and I got up and found her in the living room. She was extremely agitated and we tried to console her, to no avail. Soon she was calling us names, screaming, and trying to hit and kick us as we attempted to subdue her.

We ended up taking her down and Sara again sat across the back of her thighs and restrained her arms as Jenny raged. She swore at us, spit, clawed, and kicked her feet as she tried to break free.

I got my first taste of restraining her when I relieved Sara as her strength was waning. It amazed me how strong our seven-year-old daughter was, and I flashed to how I had always heard that people with mental illness could pull on massive reserves of strength as they raged. Jenny's small,

Asian body had developed thick muscles and, while shorter than most kids her age, her strength was impressive.

I continued restraining her for about twenty minutes and she showed no sign of letting up. Sara called a local psychiatric hospital and told them we would be bringing Jenny in. We woke Andrew, and somehow got all of us in the car. Sara sat with Jenny in the backseat and had to twice stop her from trying to open the door as we drove the four miles to the hospital.

By the time we arrived, it was after 3:00 a.m. Jenny had begun to deescalate and the charming side of her personality was ramping up. She even made the admitting nurse laugh as she questioned Jenny about what had been going on.

A psychiatrist examined her and, by 5:00 a.m., determined she was all right. He said there was no reason to keep her and wrote up her discharge. We trudged to the car and Jenny fell asleep as we drove the short distance back to the house.

I carried Jenny in and placed her in bed. Sara and I looked at one another after we had tucked Andrew back in bed and returned to our room.

"Can you believe her?" Sara said, a tired smile breaking across her face. "She charmed the nurses and doctor like nothing had happened."

"It's amazing how quickly she can go from raging to being the cute little Asian girl everyone adores," I said. "You don't ever know where it is going. But one thing's for sure. It's never boring around here."

Sara agreed. We could never gauge what we were going to get—the charming little girl whose manners were second to none or the raging kid whose anger was so great she would bite, claw, curse, kick, spit, and hit for no apparent reason.

What made it even more exasperating was that we rarely knew what would set her off. We lived on edge for the next couple of months. There were a few more instances of needing to restrain her. When she calmed down, she became a sobbing puddle of a kid in my lap, apologizing for her behavior and often wondering aloud why she acted as she did.

As the winter ended, Jenny seemed more agitated than normal and her oppositional behavior reached a new level. We were struggling to control her and took her to a psychiatric hospital in Milwaukee, where they admitted her, after a long night of restraint and wrestling in our living room. They evaluated her and kept her overnight. The admitting doctor's preliminary diagnosis was obsessive-compulsive disorder. He added the possibility of oppositional/defiant disorder and prescribed Prozac for her.

When we went to visit the next day, the nurse who had administered the first dose of meds told us that an hour after Jenny had received the Prozac, she'd come to the nurse's station and asked for another one of "those little green and yellow pills."

That was so Jenny.

She remained in the hospital for the next few days, and we talked several times with the doctor who followed her. In addition to his initial diagnosis, he wondered if Jenny was having any issues with being adopted.

Sara and I never felt it was a problem, but we were open to most anything if it would help. Sara discovered a local therapist who specialized in adoption therapy. She did a comprehensive evaluation after we met with her and Jenny saw her. She concluded that Jenny had no issues with being adopted and, in fact, had strongly bonded with us.

The pattern for Jenny's young life had been established. It mirrored the roller-coaster ride we had experienced with Sara's cancer. We were learning, firsthand, about the ups and downs of mental illness. What was different was the intensity of it all. Jenny's disorder created a massive level of stress, something we didn't experience with Sara's illness.

Sara's working time at the state hospital in Pueblo was now of even greater benefit. Fortunately, she had seen children and adolescents. It gave us a great foundation from which we would manage, as best we could, Jenny's aberrant behavior.

It is vastly different, though, when it is your child. Sara had treated some of the most severely disturbed kids in Colorado. These were children who had often been abused and went on to commit assault or murder, abuse animals, sexually abuse others, and/or commit arson. When Sara was six months pregnant with Andrew, one of her female patients had become so enraged over some inconsequential matter that she came at Sara and kicked her in the stomach. Fortunately, there was no injury, but it reinforced just how truly sick these kids were.

We were able to manage Jenny pretty well but she had flare-ups about every eight to nine months. Almost a year after Jenny's first hospital stay, Sara and I scheduled a meeting with a psychologist who had seen Jenny for an evaluation. He was set to walk us through his treatment plan, and we drove to his office for a 7:00 p.m. meeting.

Andrew had agreed to watch his sister. We always made a point of ensuring that Andrew knew he did not have to watch her. We asked this night if he would be willing to do so and he was fine with it.

Sara and I were about halfway through our session when her cell phone rang. It was Elena, our neighbor. She and her husband, Mike, who I worked with at Miller, were the closest friends we had in Wisconsin. Elena said everything was fine but that she had Jenny at their house. She had gone to our home after Andrew called and told her that Jenny was out of control. He had been somewhat frantic and asked Elena if she would come over right away to help him. She hurried across the street and found Andrew holed up in his room. She discovered Jenny in her room, playing and acting as if nothing had happened.

Elena went into Andrew's room and found him pretty shaken over what had occurred. Apparently, Jenny was unhappy with the fact her brother would not play a game with her. As was often the case in his middle school years, he had been in his room, doing homework. Jenny had badgered him to play, even though Andrew told her he had schoolwork to do, and he finally closed the door and locked it so she could not get in.

Her solution was to get a hammer and bang on Andrew's door. She pounded with such force that she put a hole in it.

Sara and I hurried home and found Elena waiting with a calm Jenny. As was often the case after such an episode, she was so calm and seemed so normal it was difficult to believe she was the same kid who, just minutes before, had been so out of control. Andrew was all right, just shaken by the fact that Jenny had actually done what she had.

Life continued rolling along for us. Lost in all the drama with Jenny was the fact there was no sign of a cancer recurrence for Sara. Our day-to-day existence, outside of Jenny's outbursts, had become nearly normal.

However, that would change before long.

CHAPTER
6

As the adventures comprising our life continued flying our way, I was contacted by an executive recruiter about a job in the Detroit area. At Miller, things were fine but I was becoming bored.

The position was vice president of communications for Championship Auto Racing Teams, the leading IndyCar racing sanctioning organization. I would be back in sports, which was something I missed, and it offered significantly more income. I accepted the new challenge and started in December. As we had done when we moved from Denver, Sara and the kids remained in Wisconsin until Andrew and Jenny completed school. We moved into our home in the Detroit suburbs in June of 1997.

Jenny continued her ups and downs, and Sara did her usual excellent job of keeping our family on track while I was away. Jenny had another flare-up before we moved but we figured we would get settled in the Detroit area and become connected with some good psychiatric practitioners who would be able to help us.

For the first time in our married life, Sara's job search did not land her in the position she wanted right away. She worked in home health initially but persevered and ended up doing what she wanted—serving as a contract therapist for Troy schools, the district Andrew and Jenny attended.

One of the benefits of Sara's work was her access to a variety of people who could help with Jenny. We took advantage of those contacts to get Jenny connected with psychologists, therapists, social workers, and others who could help us figure out what it was we were up against.

The first couple of years in Troy, life went along pretty much as it had in Wisconsin. For the most part, our life had settled back into somewhat of a routine. We built a small circle of friends and saw our families semi-frequently. It was great to be so close to my parents and Sara's mom. Also, my three brothers and sister were within two hours' drive, and Sara's youngest sister's home fell within that radius as well. It was great that Andrew and Jenny had the opportunity to spend a good amount of time getting to better know their cousins.

As always, a significant piece of moving included locating doctors, with an emphasis on finding an oncologist with whom Sara was comfortable. She checked around and ended up at Cancer Care Associates (CCA) with Dr. David Decker, the lead doctor in the practice. It was affiliated with a massive hospital system, William Beaumont, located in Royal Oak. CCA was one of the the best practices in metro Detroit and had a terrific reputation.

Fortunately, as the late nineties unfolded, Sara's visits were only for follow-ups—regular blood work, an occasional X-ray, and a couple annual scans. Otherwise, our thoughts about cancer had slipped into the back of the closet.

It was a long and welcomed respite from the two bouts we had previously experienced.

Unfortunately, round three lurked on the horizon.

When you live in Michigan, winter is, to say the least, bleak. The gray days far outnumber those in which you catch a glimpse of the sun. From November through March, one word serves as the primary descriptor: dreary. The people who run the schools recognize that fact and allow for a winter break every year. Fortunate families overwhelm the Detroit Airport in mid-February and head off to warmer climes in Florida, Mexico, or Arizona. As 1999 wound down, we made the choice to spend our winter break in Tucson.

Tucson's sunshine and warm temperatures found us spending much of our week outdoors. Jenny couldn't get enough of the pool and I even coaxed Andrew into playing golf. Much to his dismay. We also spent time riding horses in the desert, visiting the Sonora Desert Museum, and exploring a cave southeast of town used by late nineteenth century desperados to hide out after robbing banks.

Jenny's bizarre behavior reared its head a couple times and there was a day when Sara told Andrew and me to go off and do something while she and Jenny wrestled with her illness at the hotel. The noise level became greater than it should have a few times, and I was concerned hotel management might intervene. Fortunately they didn't.

As the week passed, Sara showed signs of not feeling well. She was always a master at concealing when she was physically off her game. It reached a peak, though, when we toured the Sonora Desert Museum. Sara excused herself for a period of time to go to the ladies room, where I later learned, she vomited several times. I had an uneasy feeling about it when she returned to continue the tour and I asked how she was doing.

"I must be getting the flu," she said. She looked pale and weak and I was concerned. "It's not a big deal," she said. "I'll be fine in a day or two."

A few days after our return to Michigan Sara mentioned that a couple of people had commented on her tan and how good she looked. I had noticed how she had taken on a deep brown color that was almost copper. It made her look like a woman who had spent the entire week by the pool. She had always tanned deeply, a reflection of her brown eyes and dark brunette hair, and I thought little more of it.

The week continued and she still felt under the weather. Also, she had begun itching and told me she thought maybe she had gotten something from her kids at school. A few students had recently been diagnosed with scabies. It was one of the downsides of working as a school therapist.

That Saturday morning, as we roused ourselves, my first look at Sara told me that something was definitely wrong. Her brown irises were no longer ringed by white. That part of her eye was a pool of bright yellow.

"Your eyes . . . the whites are yellow," I said in a voice that was a bit panicky.

Suddenly, we had another thing for our Saturday to-do list. In fact, this had quickly moved to the top.

"How do you feel? We need to call Dr. Khilanani right away and find out what's going on with this," I said as Sara scrambled to get out of bed and bolted to the bathroom to look in the mirror.

I stood behind her as she peered into the giant glass that filled one wall.

"It's jaundice," she said and she started to cry. "This isn't good. The cancer's back. I bet it's in my liver and that's why I'm jaundiced," she said, her voice trailing off as she began to sob. "This explains why I have felt so crappy the last week and a half."

I held her tightly as that longtime missing, but all too familiar, sense of dread bubbled up in my stomach. I felt a little nauseous and my brain began to race. The awful feeling that meant cancer was in our lives had returned.

Indeed. It's back, I thought.

I called our doctor and her service answered. I explained the situation to the woman who answered, trying to maintain a sense of calm as I did.

"I'll let them know. The doctor on call will be back with you shortly," she said in a calm and pleasant voice. The phone rang in about twenty minutes. After a brief description of Sara's symptoms, he told us to immediately go to the Beaumont Hospital Emergency Room where Sara would be evaluated.

We showered and dressed quietly. We always seemed to get quiet in these situations as we processed where we were. I had learned over the years that I best dealt with adversity when I suppressed my emotions in situations like this, focusing my thoughts on being logical and rational. I was proud of the fact that I was able to do so. It was a strategy that, for me, was not much different than counting to ten, taking a deep breath, and then determining next steps.

I broke the silence by saying I would get Andrew up and tell him we needed to go to the doctor—staying away from the "hospital" word to avoid raising unnecessary alarm—and we would need him to watch Jenny.

Andrew agreed to look after Jenny and asked if his mother was okay. I could see concern in his eyes and on his face. He knew. As I turned to leave the room, he asked if it was the cancer.

"We don't know, Andrew. But we'll find out and, like always, we'll do what we have to do."

The drive to the hospital was a short one. The admitting nurse had been notified by the on-call doctor that we were coming. After the required paperwork, we went into an exam room and waited. We held hands and stared into the white wall as we sat in chairs adjacent to one another.

The ER doc was a relatively young woman who was smiling as she greeted us. "So, tell me why you're here this morning," she said, looking through the chart that answered the question she had just asked.

Sara offered her story and I joined in as needed.

"Let's get some blood work started. That will give us a better idea of what's going on."

We returned to the waiting room after the blood draw and waited, anxious to know, but fully anticipating results that were less than favorable. After what seemed like an eternity, a nurse called us back to the exam room. The doctor returned a few moments later.

"We have the results," she said, "and we need to get you on some medication right away. I'm afraid your bilirubin is quite elevated. The normal level is .5; your results came back slightly over 20."

The cause of her liver being incapacitated was not yet determined. But we felt in our guts that it was the return of her cancer. If there were tumors in her liver, the result could very well be the flu-like symptoms and itching Sara had experienced the past two weeks.

"We need to run a couple of scans to determine what is up with your liver, to see what is causing it to no longer work as it should," the ER doctor said.

A CT scan was scheduled and we moved to the radiology department where we waited an unusually short time before Sara was summoned for the test. She returned about forty-five minutes later and we were back home by noon.

"We always knew this could happen. I just never thought it would," Sara said as tears welled in her eyes. The cancer had remained in remission from 1989 until 2000.

Sara's oncologist had voiced reservations about her being on the Tamoxofin since we had arrived in Troy. He was worried about the side effects of taking the drug for as long as she had. Since it came out of clinical trials in the late eighties, there had been a smattering of research about long-term impact. The concern was always about how it could affect liver function. Dr. Decker had made the decision to take her off it in late 1997, and we had reluctantly agreed with his decision.

Our fear now was that her breast cancer had metastasized to her liver. The scan would tell us.

I wondered where all this would end up. It was so easy to get mired in the negativity of it all. But that, I kept telling myself, served no constructive purpose. There was no benefit in going there. I tried my best to remain positive. And the numbness that came with these episodes was returning. I kept telling myself that we'd had eleven consecutive cancer-free years—good years for Sara, the kids, and me. It could have been much worse, I thought.

Unfortunately, as we were about to discover, the good years were coming to an end.

We met with Dr. Khilanani Monday morning. The CT scan results lay atop the stack of files containing the story of Sara's health over the last several years.

"Your bilirubin number is not good," she said in her usual, straight-forward manner. "And the scan shows that your liver has tumors of various sizes. They have caused your liver to shut down and the result is this high bilirubin number. It was good you got on the medications as you did, when you did."

She sighed as she looked at the four manila folders stuffed with paperwork that reached more than nine inches tall. She seemed to be summoning the courage to tell us something we probably would not like hearing. She took a deep breath and then spoke.

"I have to tell you . . . because of your symptoms and history, your insurance may not agree to cover treatment for you."

Dr. Khilanani's husband shared space in the Troy Beaumont Professional Building. He provided care to hundreds as an oncologist. That knowledge base allowed her to know and understand much more about cancer than the average family practice physician.

"You know I will do all I can to help move this along, but you should get with your oncologist as soon as possible to see what he recommends," she added, offering a genuine degree of sympathy. "I didn't want to bring it up, but we have always been honest and forthright with one another. I believe it's important that you understand what you are up against."

We did understand what we were up against. This was very serious. It is deadly serious when your liver is so diseased it won't work. We understood.

"We'll get with Dr. Decker right away," I said as Sara was getting out of the paper gown and back into her jeans and sweater.

We were silent as we walked to the car, but finally spoke as we headed home.

"Well, it can't be much worse, can it? But then, I guess it always can be worse, can't it?"

"Yes," I said, trying to be the positive one while Sara wrestled with the news. "It could be worse. I always think about how long we've had since you were first diagnosed. Then it doesn't seem as daunting."

"I know," Sara said. "But you know how I feel about chemo, and I'm certain this will end up there. It's the last resort. It kills the cancer. But it also kills good cells. It attacks your immune system. I was hopeful that I would never have to do it. It's symbolic of a stage I hoped we would never reach."

"Well at least we have it as an option. We can't forget that it's been seventeen years since this all started. We could have been facing chemo a long time ago."

Silence returned as I mentally paged through the years that had elapsed since that fateful day in 1983. My long flight from Toronto to Denver seemed a lifetime ago.

Sara had her cell phone in hand and called Dr. Decker's office to make an appointment. After she explained the situation, there was a pause, and then she started talking again.

"Thanks for getting me in so quickly," she said. "We'll be right over."

In times like this, the healthcare system can be amazingly efficient.

CHAPTER

7

Beaumont is a massive city hospital, one of the largest in the country, with more than a thousand beds. One of the longtime misconceptions held by many about southeast Michigan is that it is a vast, crime ridden wasteland that has never recovered from the 1967 Detroit riots. While the city itself has areas that are scary and very challenged, many of the suburbs rank among some of the best living in the country. When we moved to Oakland County in 1997, it was one of the top ten most affluent counties in America.

As the auto industry was flying high, Detroit developed a formidable infrastructure to support the many needs of an advanced and healthy culture. The arts, education, and high-end shopping thrived. In the 1990s, and into the early part of the next decade, life was very good—until the automotive downturn caused tax rates to erode, people to move away, and much of the climate of the area to change dramatically.

Beaumont is one of the foundational elements of the Detroit area healthcare infrastructure. However, for all its great staff and healthcare advances, the facility is often best remembered as the hospital where Dr. Jack Kevorkian dropped individuals who had sought his assistance to end their lives.

The large, eight-sided fish tank sitting in the middle of the waiting room at Cancer Care's Beaumont Royal Oak campus always fascinated me. It provided distraction from the stark and, many times, deadly realities that hung over the room. I found it interesting that you could stare into a fish tank for a long time and see nothing.

I surveyed the faces in the room. A couple were tearstained. A few more offered a veneer of false hope. The vast majority, though, looked tired. Very tired. Fish-tank stares, I thought. You could tell the patients who were seriously ill by their sunken eyes and grayish skin tone. The waiting room was the last buffer between the relative normalcy of the real world and the often surreal scenes encountered in cancer examination rooms.

We were called and followed the nurse to Dr. Decker's exam room. He was a wonderful man, one who genuinely cared and had become a good friend. He always wanted to absorb all he could about each patient and case. And he took the time, as best he could, to get to know those he counseled. We waited a few minutes before he tapped on the door and strolled in. As always, his lab coat was bright-white and heavily starched, his name embroidered on the left chest.

"Dr. Khilanani called me. She wanted me to have the details of the case immediately because she knew you would be seeing me as quickly as you could," he said, peering over the straight-line frame of his reading glasses.

As she often did in a situation with her physicians, Sara took the initiative to open the conversation. She described how she felt while we were in Arizona and how it had continued since our return.

"I had a look at the CT scan and your liver has several tumors in it," he said. "It's understandable why it has basically shut down.

"Chemo is the course of treatment for you," he added, matter-of-factly, without looking up from the chart.

Sara wondered what the other options might be.

"With the tumors as diffuse as they are, surgery isn't a viable option," Dr. Decker said. "And radiation won't work quickly enough. You can't go on with your bilirubin count as high as it is. We need immediate results. Chemo is the best approach," he reiterated in the commonsense tone we didn't want to hear, but genuinely appreciated.

I chimed in, bringing up the question sitting heavy on our minds.

"David," I said. "Dr. Khilanani brought up that our insurance may not pay for the treatment because of the symptoms and what the lab work shows. Can they do that?"

We didn't know the exact cost of the drug but knew it was prohibitively expensive. Several thousand dollars for each infusion.

He sat silently for a few moments as he considered what I had said and then offered, "Obviously, I don't know what they'll do, but don't worry about it. Even if they do deny payment, we will take care of it."

A sense of relief fell over us. Sara and I knew David well enough that his word was all we needed. And we knew she would get the best care they could provide.

That was a good thing. She would need it.

I thought of an old adage we had often considered in our cancer battle: "If the cancer doesn't kill you, the cure probably will." It was often made in jest. But when you are dealing with chemotherapy, you discover just how true that statement is.

The chemicals pumped into your body do not discriminate. Sure, they kill the cancer. But they also knock out your good cells. And your immune system can begin to severely deteriorate. In Sara's case, the drug prescribed by Dr. Decker was Taxol. It was initially found in the bark of the Pacific yew tree but, by the time it was administered to Sara, it was manufactured synthetically.

Natural or synthetic, it is an extremely potent and powerful cell killer. Sara had done her usual research and was apprehensive about its effects as we again sat in the waiting room at Cancer Care a couple of days after Dr. Decker's assessment.

Sara despised being sick. Until her breast cancer, she had always been healthy, active, and vibrant. She knew the chemo would sap her energy to a level that would not allow her to do near what she was used to doing.

One of the nurses came into the waiting room and told us they were ready for us in the infusion center. We followed her. The place where patients received the drugs through IVs was an area of eight burgundy leather, reclining chairs. Many were already occupied, even though it was barely 8:00 a.m. Each had its own station, separated from the other chairs by sliding white curtains. Televisions were positioned between the stations, two chairs sharing a screen. We walked past this area to a more private room that was physically separated from the others. We sat down and a nurse came in soon after. We assumed they put newcomers to the chemo process in the separate room.

"I will be bringing the Taxol in soon and we can get started," she said. "I need to finish mixing it and will be right back."

She walked out and into a small room two doors down. It was at the end of the hall and almost closet-like. My curiosity got the best of me and I stepped into the doorway and looked up the hall. The nurse put on a pair of safety glasses and then gowned up in a rubber apron and rubber gloves. It was only after taking on this mad scientist aura did she begin to mix the drug and move it into the IV bag. The irony of the lengths she went to in order to avoid getting the drug on her, as well as keeping it sterile, really hit home.

Wow, I thought. No way did she want any of it on her, but it was going to be pumped into Sara's body. I wondered about Sara's ability to handle it. A sense of anxiety and fear washed over me.

Way serious stuff.

I helped Sara get settled in her infusion chair, tuned the television to the channel she wanted, and reminded her I had to head to the office. With all her recent appointments and tests, I hadn't been able to keep up with things at work.

"I know you're busy. I'll be okay," she said with a weak smile as I leaned in to give her a hug and kiss.

"I'll be back in a few hours. You have your cell phone, right? Just call and let me know what's up," I said.

I drove to my office and settled in to try to catch up on an ever growing pile of work. One of many ongoing caregiver pressures revolves around the stress of being absent from work. Trying to find a balance that allowed me to continue doing what was expected at work and devoting the time I needed to care for Sara was a never-ending juggling act. I was fortunate to have a boss who was very supportive, but I regularly felt the stress of having so many balls in the air. I tried to focus on the tasks at hand, but my mind wandered to Sara and her first chemo treatment on several occasions. I was plowing through the stack of work when the phone on my desk came to life. It had been an hour and a half since I left Sara at Beaumont and my caller ID indicated the call was from her.

I picked up and heard Sara's cracking voice. She, I could immediately tell, was trying to maintain her composure.

"They started the treatment and within five minutes, I had such horrible back spasms, they had to stop it," she said, starting to cry.

It quickly became obvious where I needed to be, and I started putting files away as I listened to her.

"They're now trying to decide what to do. What if I can't tolerate this?"

"We'll figure it out. I'll be there as quickly as I can," I told her, trying to be calm and assuring.

I called my CEO's assistant and told her I was going to have to leave again. While the people at CART had been supportive and told me to take the time I needed, I felt my stress level rising as I thought of how I was getting further behind with each hour away from the office. The racing season was less than a month off and I had a ton of things on my plate.

But Sara needed me and that was the priority.

I headed back to Cancer Care and when I got there, the receptionist acknowledged my presence right away. She looked concerned and immediately went for the nurse.

"I'm so glad you're here," the nurse said as she approached. Her tone was serious. "We moved Sara to the hospital, the seventh floor. She's been admitted and will be getting her treatment there. Her back spasms were so painful we couldn't continue the treatment here as planned. We'll give her the Taxol much more slowly than usual. It could take the rest of the day."

I looked at my watch and saw it was not yet 11:00 a.m.

"We have so many patients scheduled here at the infusion center and can't tie up a chair for the entire day," she continued, taking on an apologetic tone. "In the hospital, she'll be able to take the infusion at the rate she needs. Hopefully, that will allow us to avoid the spasms. And they have better access to the drugs they might need to keep Sara comfortable."

I wondered if this development would affect her ability to be treated on an ongoing basis and voiced this to the nurse. She didn't think it would, adding that patients typically build a tolerance to the drug that allows them to take it faster.

I thanked her, turned, and left. I slowly began my walk through the Beaumont complex to the seventh floor—the cancer floor. We knew of it, but Sara had never actually been admitted. The fact that we had taken another step down the cancer road was not lost on me.

I found Sara lying in bed, her head raised to forty-five degrees. An IV line was attached to her left arm.

"I'm so glad you got here," she said, smiling weakly. Her eyes were swollen and red. "The pain was unbelievable. I've never experienced anything like it. They gave me some muscle relaxants and it is okay now, but I'm so sore."

"I'm sorry this started out this way," I said.

It had been difficult enough to get mentally prepared for the chemo. Knowing Sara needed this powerful drug to stay alive was stressful enough, but this development took her treatment in a direction we could never have expected.

"When I talked to the nurse at Dr. Decker's office, she said this is unusual but it does happen sometimes," I added. "She said you'll build a tolerance and it will become easier to take it as you go along."

I sat next to her bed and we engaged in casual conversation for about a half hour. A nurse came by twice during that time, providing some comfort to both Sara and me. Sara looked knowingly at me and, while I knew she would rather not say it, told me to go back to work. I needed the assurance that she was okay with me leaving before I could go.

I returned to the office and worked until five. Andrew returned home from Athens High School and was looking after his sister. I explained that Mom was okay, but the treatment was taking longer than expected. They assured me they would be fine, I ordered them a pizza, and headed back to Beaumont. Sara sat in the bed, IV still inserted in her arm.

We watched the liquid slowly drip down the IV line and the Taxol bag finally emptied around 7:00 p.m. It had been nearly twelve hours since we arrived at Cancer Care. Treatment No.1 was finally complete.

Sara moved slowly as she began to dress. Her back was very sore and sensitive. I helped her pull on her clothes and shoes. I wondered how her body would respond to the toxic chemicals they had pumped into her. The vision of the nurse pulling on the rubber apron and gloves popped back into my head. Serious stuff, indeed, I thought again.

"What a long day," Sara said, with a sigh as we drove home.

It was hard to see her as she was. Her eyes were red and sunken and I noticed lines in her face I had never before seen.

This was a Sara I hadn't seen in the thirty-four years I had known her.

"I'm just happy it's over. I have seven more treatments to go," she said, thinking ahead to her next session. "I can do this, but it has to get better than this."

I assured her it would, adding that we didn't have other options.

Sara sighed as she said, "I know." Her head turned toward me and she said, "I love you. Thanks for being here for me."

"I love you too," I said, as I tried to swallow the lump in my throat.

The ensuing weeks passed quickly. I was busy with my auto racing work, preparing for the 2000 season. Sara was pre-occupied with keeping herself healthy. The drug was as brutally potent as we had expected. It compromised her immune system in a devastating way.

The side effects were pretty much as advertised: a loss of appetite and a metallic aftertaste that never disappeared. Aching joints. Mouth sores. And hair loss.

Sara was never a vain woman. She didn't dote too much on makeup, hairstyles, nails, or facials. But she always looked terrific. She was fortunate that the essence of her look came from a natural beauty that didn't require a huge investment of time or beauty products. Perhaps her most striking feature was her gleaming, dark brown hair. It combined with her brown eyes in a way that drew me to her and was almost always something noticed by people she met.

We had fully anticipated her hair loss. But it was the one element of chemo's side effects that Sara most dreaded. She could deal with the joint pain. The loss of appetite was manageable. She often ate canned mandarin oranges because, for some reason, they were one of the few foods that didn't have a metallic taste to them. I bought those little cans by the case. But her hair. I knew it would be the most traumatic part of her bout with chemo—and it was.

"Look!" Sara said one morning a few days after her first treatment. She'd been in the shower, but the bathroom door flew open three or four minutes after I heard the water begin. Sara stood there, naked and dripping wet, frantically calling out for me to come into the bathroom. She had a hairbrush in her right hand and was running it through her hair. The long brunette strands were dripping wet and water was puddling under her on the bathroom tiles.

"My hair! It's falling out in clumps."

She was right. Each stroke of the brush pulled more strands from her head. Soon she was sobbing and much of her hair was pulled from her scalp and lying in the bathroom sink.

"I knew it would happen," she said between sobs as I held her wet body in my arms. "But I didn't think it would be like this. All of it coming out at once? I can't believe it."

I just held her, knowing that there was nothing I could say that would provide comfort. This was one of those "just being there" moments that would become a crucial and frequent part of our lives over the next several years. I had to be strong and not offer more than a shoulder and my hugs.

"You're right," I said after several minutes had passed and she calmed down a bit. "We knew this was coming. I know it rings pretty hollow right now, but it will grow back."

Her brown eyes focused in on me like a pair of lasers. I flashed back to the thought of not saying too much and kept my thoughts to myself. I helped her dry off and she got dressed.

Sara had thought long and hard about the hair loss scenario. In her naturally creative way, she planned an alternative that was cute and simple, but did not shy away from the fact she was bald.

She had purchased baseball caps in several colors. They were the kind with soft, head-hugging, unstructured fronts that allowed the cap to contour her head. She would match her outfit to one of the caps and then place a scarf around the base of the cap, covering the top of her ears. It solved the problem in a fashionable way.

"I think it looks pretty good," she said as she sized herself up through eyes that had been filled with tears a few minutes earlier. "I'll remove the rest of my hair—if there is any left—when I shower tomorrow. I know we expected this, but the reality of it just came crashing down on me in the shower. I'm sorry. I just lost it when it happened."

"It's okay," I said as I held her again. "If the chemo helps as it's supposed to, losing your hair is a small price to pay. And your cap and scarf look great."

Her familiar spunk and focus had returned, if even momentarily. You expect side effects when you deal with cancer. What was less expected were the residual effects of the disease. They often are every bit as devastating—and sometimes even more so—than the physical challenges.

Sara had taken a leave from her job and as the chemo regime unfolded, she had kept the Troy schools in the know about her illness. The administration and staff were very supportive and regularly checked in for updates about Sara's condition and progress. We knew, though, that the Taxol's potency would eventually wreak havoc on Sara's immune system. And, in working with kids who were constantly getting colds, the flu, and who knows what else, it was going to become difficult for her to continue working.

We met with Dr. Decker for a routine checkup before Sara's second treatment and confronted him with the issue of Sara's ability to work.

"I advise against it," he said. "You have to focus your energy on getting well. Let's not forget just how sick you were. While your condition is slowly improving, that could very easily change if you come in contact with a cold or flu. You have to be careful to avoid pneumonia."

We knew he was right. Sara asked if he thought she might be able to return to work after she concluded the chemo and her immunity had improved.

"Let's take this a step at a time," he said. "You really do need to focus on the treatments and keeping yourself as strong as you can."

As Sara was getting dressed, I stepped out of the exam room and chased down Dr. Decker. Being the pragmatist I am, I asked him about Sara eventually receiving disability.

"I think, in the longer term and with her prognosis, it's probably not going to be difficult for her to get Social Security disability benefits," he said. "When the time comes, I will write a letter that should ensure that it happens. We regularly do it for patients."

Sara knew me well enough to figure out that I was up to something, and as we left the building she asked me what I had discussed with Dr. Decker.

"We talked about the potential of you getting Social Security Disability," I said, matter-of-factly.

I knew Sara so well and anticipated what she was thinking. Her dedication to her career and patients always took precedence.

"I know this is going to be tough," she said, "but I don't want to apply for disability until I absolutely have to. I want to continue working when I'm feeling better and able to do so."

"I understand," I said, trying to maintain a sense of empathy but looking at the situation objectively. "But we have lost your income in the short-term and we don't know if you will be able to work again. I think it's something we should look into."

Sara turned toward me and said, "I love my work so much. Those kids need me. I understand we need the money, but applying for disability will feel like I am conceding that I won't work again. I don't know that I'm ready for that."

I paused before I spoke, employing my best empathy skills. "I can't imagine how that feels. All I'm saying is, I think we should be prepared for it."

It was an inevitability. I wanted us to be prepared to move forward on it when Sara could no longer work. It would be a relatively small but welcome piece of financial support. The issue of finances and income were always near the forefront of my thinking. While insurance covered a good amount of her treatments, tests, and office visits, there were constant co-pays and deductibles that ate away at our savings and monthly cash flow. And then there were those instances where there was no coverage.

One of the issues that had bothered Sara since her diagnosis in 1983 was that she did not have any life insurance. Of course, with her illness and diagnosis, the insurance people had no interest in covering her.

Upon our move to Detroit, Sara met an insurance man through our church. There had been no evidence of cancer since 1989 and, in 1998, an insurance company considered her case and came back saying they were willing to cover her. She was so happy and proud of the fact that she had tracked down a policy.

The years passed and she had faithfully made the premium payments. As things were unfolding with her cancer—and the realities of our life were settling in—Sara began looking into her insurance policy and the possibilities if she were to die. She uncovered a possible solution termed a viatical settlement. She sought out a company that specialized in such agreements to see if they would be interested in working with her.

They reviewed Sara's case and agreed to purchase the policy benefit from the insurance company. They determined they would give her roughly $55,000, paid in increments over a two-year period. That was on a $100,000 death benefit. The organization obviously hoped Sara would die sooner rather than later. They would then get their money. Essentially, it was no different than placing a bet.

In her independent way, Sara went forward with the settlement without consulting me. While the money came in handy as the months passed, the reality was that I always felt we would have benefited more had we kept the policy.

They lived up to the agreement, giving us the money as they indicated they would. It just seemed like we ended up on the short end of the stick.

In the end, Sara would beat the odds. She lived long enough that the company appeared to have lost money, at least on paper.

The financial piece of her illness was only beginning to manifest itself. We were joining the growing ranks of people whose lives strained under the weight of healthcare costs.

Another side effect of cancer.

Sara continued with her Taxol treatments. She was admitted to the hospital for her second and third go-rounds and the back spasms diminished. Of course, the misery of a compromised immune system, the metallic taste that never went away, the aching joints, the hair loss, the occasional nausea, and the general malaise all combined to make her life far less than a cakewalk.

These were all legitimate and very real reasons for negativity to creep into Sara's life. Many would say she was entitled to that negativity. However, she almost always kept her focus positive, continually falling back to her position of being the best patient she could be.

That doesn't mean it was easy.

Life with cancer is a never-ending world of anticipation. Unfortunately, it's not the kind of anticipation you have as a child waiting for Christmas morning. Instead, it is a gnawing sensation, a feeling in the pit of your stomach that the other shoe will drop. You don't know when. You don't know how. And you most likely will never know why. But the underlying feeling remains: there is more to come. When will it arrive?

The Beaumont cancer ward became a second home for us. It was staffed by some of the most wonderful people in the world, people whose level of professionalism is rivaled only by their compassion. The nurses were always busy, yet ready to offer a caring smile, a kind word, or a touch to a hand or forearm conveying the love they had for patients and their families, as well as their work. It was a bustling place of radiology doctors and technicians, oncologists, occupational and speech therapists, neurologists, endocrinologists, and, of course, nurses.

Underlying that feeling of activity, though, was a sense of uneasiness on the parts of patients and their families. Anyone who has been or is in this situation knows what I'm talking about. Patients and their families understand the magnitude of the situations they often face. And it's visible—an expression of the churn that is going on inside everyone touched by the disease. The appearance of a pastor, priest, or rabbi always reinforces the seriousness of the environment and is a vivid reminder of where this could end up.

Cancer has a way of grabbing your attention and not letting go. The reality is that, while advances occur every day, the disease seems to be as smart as those thousands who spend their life's work trying to eradicate it.

There's a lot of looking out windows, staring at walls, and mindless television watching on the cancer floor. There are so many questions and so many things to consider, yet there are never enough answers. Even children understand the seriousness of it. When they visit, their usual carefree manner evaporates within a few minutes of their arrival as the realization of life's more difficult side sweeps over them.

From the get-go, we talked long and hard about the best way to inform the kids of Sara's illness. It was a real challenge because we wanted to walk a fine line between providing enough information to make them feel they were in the know, but not so much that they became overwhelmed, scared, or confused by the facts. We generally followed the tact of conveying the basics and then waited for questions. We were often surprised by their ability to grasp what was going on, as well as the gravity of the situation. And their questions often indicated an insight that was unexpectedly deep and thoughtful.

Andrew was in his senior year of high school when Sara's disease metastasized to her liver. He had a profound understanding of the situation. From a young age, he tended to be a bit of a worrier. We knew there was little we had to explain to him.

"Will this cancer thing make Mom die?" he asked me one day when he and I were watching a basketball game. "Does she have a good chance against it?"

I hesitated because I did not want to scare him but did want to give him an honest answer to his question.

"We really don't know what will happen, Andrew. This is one of those times in life when you just have to trust that you are doing all you can, that the doctors know what they are doing, and that it will work out for the best as we go ahead. Dr. Decker thinks Mom has a chance if she stays on her treatments and takes care of herself. We need to do our part, too. We can help by encouraging her and staying positive. The good thing is that your mom doesn't need to be encouraged much to remain positive."

I could tell there was something else simmering behind his brown eyes.

"Do you have other questions?" I asked.

"I just wonder sometimes why this happened to Mom," he said. "She cares so much, especially for the kids who are her patients. She cares so much for others who don't have much. She is such a good person, someone who will help anyone. It just doesn't seem fair."

I thought for a moment. Andrew had raised a question that had crossed my mind many times. Since he was our natural born child, it was a reasonable question. I rarely voiced it, though, knowing there was no real answer. It was one of those thoughts that could gnaw at your gut and occupy your mind in a way that was not productive.

"I wish we had answers to a lot of questions around Mom's cancer, Andrew. The reality is, we don't. And many of those questions will never be answered. While it would be nice to have answers, the reality is that when all is said and done, it doesn't really matter. Knowing doesn't change anything. We can get bogged down in the whys and hows. I believe that's wasted energy. We need all of our energy to be there for Mom."

For Jenny, it was different. She knew a small amount about her mom's illness, but she didn't really need more than we passed along. It could easily overwhelm her and, as we were finding, Jenny did not need more stimulation. In her world, most everything was best when it was black and white. Mom being sick meant Mom wasn't as available for her.

"When will she be better?" she once said. "I just want everything to be like it was before she got sick."

"I think she will be better soon," I told her. "She should start feeling better soon."

She usually accepted the minimalistic answer and moved on. After Sara's first Taxol treatment, she talked with the Cancer Care staff about having a port placed in her chest. With the ongoing infusion of chemicals, her left arm was under assault. It was beginning to look and feel like a pin cushion. Because of her radical mastectomy in 1983, it was critical for doctors and nurses to avoid using her right arm for blood draws or injections of any kind. The resulting neuropathy could render her arm less and less functional.

The port—a self-sealing, silicone rubber device with an attached plastic tube that connected to a vein—would serve as the access point for the chemotherapy. It also was used for blood draws, which were occurring more and more regularly. She arranged to have the device inserted in her chest wall in an out-patient surgical procedure at Beaumont and all went well. She was relieved to no longer need to have her arm poked and stuck.

Sara was always on the lookout for accomplished port practitioners who knew how to properly access the site. Those individuals were not rare, but their presence meant Sara's hospital or treatment center visit would go more smoothly.

As her treatments continued, Sara's immune system became less and less capable of fighting off bacteria and other germs. After the third treatment, she was told to eliminate contact with flowers and plants. They might carry germs that could infiltrate her system and deliver some illness. Her healthcare pros also told her to avoid crowds because individuals walking about with a cold or some other illness could easily infect her. We stayed home as a result.

We went to Beaumont's massive imaging center for a liver scan after her fourth treatment and, remarkably, the cancer in her liver was beginning to neutralize and recede. Her bilirubin numbers had also dropped dramatically and she was feeling considerably better, despite the fact that she was weakened by the chemotherapy.

CT and MRI machines were not in plentiful supply at that time and appointments were scheduled pretty much around the clock. As our lives swirled about in a way that didn't allow us to maintain much control, we would kid about having a "date" at 11:00 p.m. on Friday to go to Beaumont for a CT scan. We would return home at 1:00 a.m. and find the kids sound asleep. Our dogs, Allie and Murphy, greeted us with sleepy eyes but happily wagging tails.

By the first of September, Sara had completed six treatments and was looking at two more before ending the miserable monthly regime. But Sara had been feeling well and wondered if she could end the treatments early.

"Well, your numbers have been good," Dr. Decker said as he looked at the charts. "And the scans are indicating the tumors in your liver are shrinking and seem to have basically been neutralized. I would say, let's do this next treatment and do some more tests. If things continue to improve, I'd say you can consider skipping the final treatment."

Sara was pleased and I could see in her face how relieved she felt. The treatment infusions had shrunk from more than ten hours her first time around to slightly less than two hours. As we left Cancer Care after the appointment, Sara was more energized than I had seen her in months.

"Now that is really great news," she said with a huge smile as we climbed into the car. She was pleased with herself for confronting Dr. Decker with the question and coming away with a win. Any victory was big those days. It was nice to have an increased sense of control. And after being beaten down by a brutal but lifesaving drug, it felt good to know that the end of treatment was in sight. It seemed we were being given a reprieve and we were both ready for a "cancer break."

We couldn't wait for some time away from it all, but we wouldn't be getting quite the break we wanted. We were about to be faced with yet another bout with cancer. This time, Sara would be on the sidelines.

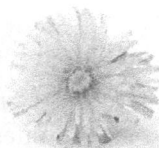

CHAPTER
8

Relief and a feeling of satisfaction flowed through me that September at the sound of Sara's voice when she called after her final Taxol treatment. Even though she had done her best to stay upbeat during the chemotherapy, the joy had been missing from her voice for some time. Fortunately, the joy had come back and was clearly audible and undeniable.

"I'm going to meet some of my friends and go to lunch," she said, sounding largely like the Sara I married in 1975. "It makes me feel so good to know this was the last treatment. I feel free again."

It was fantastic to be at a place where the treatments were behind us. As we looked back, we realized we had dodged a bullet. Sara's liver had been compromised by the cancer and we knew it had made some inroads, despite being turned back. It, indeed, felt good to know the latest episode was behind us. But the gnawing that is a side effect of cancer remained. There was always that feeling of uneasiness prompted by the fact that we knew it could return at any moment. Deep down, we knew the odds were that another dandelion would pop up. I just hoped it wouldn't be so firmly rooted that we couldn't eliminate it.

Our lives moved back to a more normal pace. Other than feeling better, the best development—certainly best from Sara's perspective—was that her hair started coming back. She initially looked like a ten-year-old boy and continued wearing her scarves and caps. As it grew in and got longer, it was darker than the brown she had for the first forty-eight years of her life and, strangely, it was curlier than before.

The kids were happy that life had reached a level of greater normalcy. Jenny had started middle school in sixth grade and seemed to be doing okay. She always had her academic struggles, but the social elements were often even more difficult for her. Her bipolar disorder caused her to sometimes behave strangely and her outbursts, visual ticks, bossiness, and difficulty in getting along impeded friendships.

For Andrew, a new chapter was about to unfold. A couple of years earlier, he had started considering colleges. He liked what he found in some, not so much in others. His propensity for causes and helping others made it difficult for him to find much value in going off to school for four more years. Andrew's academic abilities were never in question. It was a question of being true to himself, doing the right thing to help others.

That being his focus, he decided to sit out of school for a year and applied for a position with AmeriCorps, the domestic Peace Corps program established by the Clinton Administration. It was the perfect diversion for Andrew at this point in his life. While he cared deeply about his mom and family, he also needed a break from the intensity that came with Sara's cancer and Jenny's mental disorder.

After being accepted to AmeriCorps, the question was one of where he would be located. The program provided a variety of services in locations throughout the country. A few weeks after learning he was accepted into the program, he was assigned to a base in San Diego. He had to be there to begin his ten-month program in September.

After all Sara had gone through, she needed a break as well. She decided she wanted to drive with Andrew to California. I was a bit concerned about her making the trip. Her strength was largely back, but she made her decision to go before her treatments were complete. I knew, though, that she had made being able to drive across country with him a goal during her treatment, and she would do just about anything to fulfill that goal.

She and Andrew left in mid-September to make the 2,500-mile, four-day drive. It was exhausting, but they made it to San Diego the night before Andrew was to report to his team. It was difficult for Sara to leave him when he dropped her at the San Diego Airport and, we learned later, he was even more apprehensive about being there. He told us he had thought about leaving and returning to Michigan, feeling some guilt about being away from his mom as well as being out on his own for the first time, but he stuck it out and grew to love the other eleven members of his team as if they were a part of his family.

It was a big transition for Sara and me. For the first time in eighteen years, we were without him. Of course, we had Jenny and were able to focus on her and the issues that accompanied her bipolar illness. Sara was able to use her many healthcare and school contacts to secure help and services for Jenny.

I was busy with the conclusion of our racing season. It had been a tumultuous year at work. Among other things, the board had fired our CEO, the man who had hired me and for whom I had a great amount of respect. I looked forward to ending the year. The final race of the season came in October at California Speedway, east of Los Angeles. Before heading to the Detroit airport, I had arranged to have an ultrasound of my abdomen. I had seen Dr. Khilanani the previous week for my regular checkup to monitor my cholesterol. All was fine with the results of my blood work, but she reviewed my chart, paused, and then asked me a question.

"Have we ever done a scan of your liver?"

"No," I replied.

"I don't have any particular reason for asking, but I'd like to get a baseline look at it," she said. "You have been on Lipitor for quite some time and it would be good to have the scan so we can compare it to others in the future."

She was doing what she should to properly follow my cholesterol issues. It made perfect sense, so I agreed and made the appointment.

Several days later, the technician began the brief procedure, starting on my right side and then moving to my left. I didn't think much of it when she went back over the left half of my abdomen before she finished. I rose from the exam table, dressed, and headed to the airport.

A couple of days passed and the open-wheel, 225 mile-per-hour race cars were practicing on the two-mile oval. I was conducting a tour for some sponsors attending their first race and was in the middle of answering a question when my cell phone vibrated in my pocket. I excused myself for a moment to look and see who was calling. I recognized the number as Dr. Khilanani's office and worried that there was something wrong with Sara.

I fumbled to answer the phone, seeking a place where I could escape the screaming, high-pitched assault of 750-horsepower, turbocharged engines.

"Hello?" I said. "Hello?"

I could barely hear, but timing worked in my favor when a yellow flag waved and the roar of the cars subsided to a level where I could have a conversation.

"Ron? This is Dr. Khilanani."

Before she could say anything more, I asked if everything was okay with Sara.

"No, this isn't about Sara. I'm sorry to be calling you at your work, but this is important. This is about the ultrasound you had."

I hadn't considered the possibility that the call was about me and the scan I had. My stomach started to churn.

"The scan showed something in your left kidney, a mass of some kind."

She now had my full attention. I swallowed hard and responded.

"Just so I understand, there is a mass in my left kidney?"

"Yes," she said. "I've talked to the radiologist and Dr. Vora, a urologist I frequently work with. We're pretty certain by its shape, size, and consistency that it is a cancerous mass. I'm sorry to call you and tell you in this way, but this is a serious issue and one we must deal with quickly. I have always been forthright with you, and I wanted to talk with you as soon as possible."

I became a bit light-headed as I considered what I had heard and looked for a place to sit down.

"Often, this kind of cancer is what they call encapsulated," she continued. "What that means is that it's often fully contained in the organ. If it is dealt with quickly, it can be fully managed with surgery. I can't say that is the case here, but I can say you need to deal with this right away."

"Wow. I can't believe this is happening," was all I could say. I was stunned. I tried to gather my thoughts.

She is saying I have cancer? I really can't believe it.

"I made an appointment for you with Dr. Vora next week," she said.

"How can you be so sure this is cancer?" I asked.

"As often as they see these scans, the radiologist and Dr. Vora can almost be certain. I cannot say this too many times: This appears to be very serious, Ron. And you need to deal with it as quickly as you can."

My mind took off like one of the cars on the track. *This is surreal. I have cancer? I can't believe it. I don't have time for this. I need to be available for Sara and the kids and my work. I don't have time to be sick.*

"Ron? Ron?" she said, trying to regain my attention.

I snapped back and listened to her voice.

"Do you have any other questions?" she asked. "Again, I'm sorry I contacted you like this. I'll see you again next week."

When I hung up, I just stared at the phone and wondered why this was happening.

Whatever I told the group I was leading at the racetrack, they seemed to understand the call I had just completed was very important.

I headed to our at-track office, got my briefcase, and called home. Sara was there and I informed her of my conversation with Dr. Khilanani.

"It'll be okay," she said, reversing our traditional roles. "I guess it's my turn to take care of you for a while. Just like we have with my cancer, we'll deal with it and do what we need to make you better."

I was still dumbfounded. A million things were flying around in my head, and I verbalized some of it. I was suddenly faced with life as a patient, and I didn't like the feeling.

"Ron, slow down," Sara said as I began to rattle off a list of concerns, most dealing with things other than the cancer I had in my body. "It'll be okay. As we have always done, let's focus on getting you well. The rest of this will take care of itself."

She was right; I had to focus.

I had to begin thinking about what I needed to do to be the best patient I could be.

On Monday following the race weekend, I arrived at the Ontario, California, airport and was numb. As I waited to board my plane, I thought of all the difficult issues I had been through with CART the past few months, as well as the chemo treatments Sara had endured. The joy of our family vacation in Tucson seemed far in the past.

I was faced with a new personal reality and the four-hour flight would provide plenty of time for thought.

My mind went back to that Saturday morning in 1983 when I returned to Denver to be with Sara. The feelings welling up inside me felt strangely familiar. This time, though, it was decidedly different. I was the one facing surgery—and cancer.

I boarded the flight and fell into my seat. I was exhausted and hoped sleep would come easily. It usually did on flights but, this time, too much was going on in my head. In my few slow moments during the weekend, I'd spent time on the Internet, learning what I could about kidney cancer. From what I gathered, it sounded as if Dr. Khilanani had described it perfectly.

The whole thing was puzzling. Like Sara, I had no history of cancer in my family. I had largely been healthy to this point in my life. High cholesterol was my main health issue, and I would benefit from losing a few pounds. But otherwise, I was fine.

My thoughts moved to how this was playing out. Coulda. Woulda. Shoulda. Shouldn't I have sensed something? I had no symptoms. My research told me that the first signs are usually backache and blood in the urine. I felt fine. Logically—the way I normally approached most every situation—there was nothing to tip me off to this. Fortunately for me, Dr. Khilanani wanted the scan of my liver.

When I got home, Sara met me as I walked into the house. I felt a great sense of comfort just being home.

"How are you doing?" she said, her voice enveloping me with compassion and sympathy. Tears were forming in her pretty eyes.

I said nothing. We held one another for an extended period before Jenny came walking into the room.

"Are you guys okay?" she asked, scanning us with a puzzled look as we held each other.

"Hey, Jenny. How's my favorite girl?" I said, holding back tears as Sara and I broke our embrace and I leaned down and gave Jenny a hug. "What're you doing?"

"I was watching TV," she said. "Dad, are you going to be home for a while now since your races are over?"

I looked at Sara. Her eyes conveyed the sense of concern I was feeling in my gut. But the reality was that I had to try to stay composed in order to minimize the angst for the kids' sake. Sara had said nothing to them because we had decided we wanted to be together to tell them.

"Will you help me by getting my bag?" I asked Jenny.

"I guess," she said with some question in her voice. "I was wondering if you got me anything?"

The kids, especially Jenny, had become accustomed to me bringing them a gift when I returned from a significant trip. The season-ending race fell in that category and I had something for Jenny in my suitcase.

I collected my stuff and hauled it up the stairs to our bedroom. I put the two suitcases on the floor at the foot of the bed and then lifted the carry-on bag to the bed. Jenny stood just inside the door, studying my every move.

"I think I have something for you in here," I said as she looked at me and smiled. I pulled a small plastic bag from the clothes in the case.

"It's another tee shirt, isn't it?" she said in a "not that again" voice as I turned to hand her the bag.

"You need to look inside and find out," I said.

The shape of the bag gave away the fact it was not a tee shirt. She looked inside and found a stuffed animal, a small seal lion. Jenny had a large collection of stuffed animals and I always looked for something unique to add.

"This is really cute, Dad. I think I will name her Sammy," she said as she turned to head to her room. "Thank you."

"You're welcome," I replied. My mind wandered to how we would soon have to talk about something much more serious. Then my thoughts turned to Andrew and how we would have to tell him about my cancer by phone. His mom's illness had forced him to grow up more quickly than most kids, and now he had a second parent whose life was jeopardized by cancer.

My appointment with Dr. Vora was scheduled for the following morning. Things were moving so fast, it was mind-boggling.

After getting Jenny to school, Sara and I headed to Dr. Vora's office. One quick look at the other patients in the waiting room told me they were older than me—quite a lot older. I couldn't grasp belonging there, in that room, with those people.

A nurse called us in. As we sat waiting for him in his office, I surveyed the room and saw he was a graduate of the University of Michigan School of Medicine. A large, impressively framed and signed picture of him with former Michigan football coach Bo Schembechler graced the wall prominently behind his desk.

We had waited a couple more minutes when the door opened and Dr. Vora walked into the room. His olive complexion and dark hair were striking, and he spoke with a slight Indian accent.

He extended his hand, first to Sara, then to me.

"I see you're a Michigan man," I said with a nervous smile, making small talk. I told him I was a lifelong Michigan fan and shared his passion for Wolverine football.

"Coach Schembechler was a great coach, a real leader, and a terrific success," he said, a smile coming to his face. "I am a big Michigan fan, too. We'll get along well, I think."

He paused for a moment before delving into the meat of the matter at hand. "I wish we had a more pleasant subject to discuss this morning. I know Dr. Khilanani told you what we are quite certain we are up against. Let's take a look at the scan."

He placed what seemed to be a very large X-ray onto a light board on the wall next to his desk and flipped a switch. A series of images ran in rows across the large film. I was able to see what all the fuss was about for the first time. A dark oval was centered in my kidney, and it appeared to be about the size of a large grape. It certainly didn't look as menacing as it was.

"So, what do you think? Can you remove it without damaging my kidney?" I asked, looking at the screen and trying to fully understand the images. Hope filled my voice.

"Based on where the tumor is, I believe it is highly unlikely we can remove it without damaging your kidney beyond repair," he replied. "I want to get an MRI to determine exactly what we face here. The ultrasound is good technology—it discovered this mass. But an MRI will provide us with the detail we need to give us a better sense."

I studied the film on the board and Sara slipped her left hand into my right, weaving her fingers between mine. She squeezed, pushing her love for me through our joined hands.

"I suggest we get an MRI as quickly as we can and get you scheduled for surgery," he added. "This is not something to put off. We should deal with it as soon as possible. This kind of thing has a tendency to grow quickly. You are a lucky man. Had Dr. Khilanani not wanted the scan of your liver, we wouldn't have found this. It could have gone for weeks without detection, and then it would have been much more advanced."

I appreciated and understood his sentiments. But I was not feeling lucky. Despite all the churn around me, I felt fine. I wasn't quite sure what to say.

"You're the expert in this kind of thing. If that's the course you recommend, then let's move ahead," I said.

"All right," he said, reaching for the phone on the corner of his desk. "Let me get my scheduler going and we will set up an MRI as soon as possible. I will examine that scan and determine what I have to do. We'll get your surgery scheduled, too."

He spoke with his assistant and while I heard him talking, I wasn't paying attention to what he said. That numb feeling was returning again.

"This is serious, but I'm confident we have found this at a stage that makes it manageable," he concluded. "Fortunately, we are born with two kidneys, so even if I have to remove your left one, you will have full function with the right. There are thousands of people who live perfectly normal lives with one kidney. Let's get the MRI and go from there."

I asked questions about the possibility that the cancer had spread, how long I should be in the hospital, what to expect from a recovery standpoint, and whether or not I would need any follow-up treatments after surgery. As doctors do, they always couch their comments. Dr. Vora was no different.

"There are no guarantees, but with this at the stage it seems to be, I believe it's highly unlikely it has spread beyond the tumor in your kidney. You'll probably be hospitalized six to seven days, and the recovery will be longer than I suspect you would like—probably six weeks. As for any chemo or radiation, I expect the surgery will take care of this fully."

I was satisfied with his answers, although I didn't necessarily like what I heard. This truly was a major surgery. It would keep me laid up for much longer than I had hoped.

Sara and I left Dr. Vora and spent the next hour with the scheduler, who contacted facilities with MRI capabilities. She finally got me an appointment—for 2:15 a.m. on Saturday. It was incredible to think that in the northern suburbs of Detroit, a city with terrific healthcare, I would have to wait nearly four days to get a scan. My surgery was scheduled for the following Wednesday at 7:30 a.m. Eight days before Thanksgiving.

Sara asked me how I was doing as we left the hospital, and I wasn't even sure, myself. So much had happened over the last few days.

"We're cancer veterans, aren't we?" she said, a smile coming over her face as she tried to lighten the situation.

I looked at her and it struck me how good she looked. Her dark brown hair was coming back. The dark circles under her eyes, long a feature of her tired face during her chemo, were no longer present. Her skin color was coming back. It was hard to believe that just a few weeks earlier, she had been sitting in a chair at the Beaumont cancer unit in Royal Oak with Taxol being pumped into her. I thought about how much I loved her and how fortunate I was to have her at my side.

It wasn't like us to be serious for extended periods. I laughed in response to her comment.

"We do kind of have a corner on this cancer stuff, don't we?" I said, forcing a grin. "Too bad we weren't able to invest in Beaumont. At least then we could get something back for all we're putting into this place."

I dropped Sara off at home and went to the CART office, but focusing on the mundane was difficult to do. The company had always been supportive during our health issues and this time was no different. I was told CART was there for me if and when I needed them. I also was told to take the time I needed to recover, making certain I was able to adequately recover before coming back to work. I muddled my way through work, but I had the kids on my mind.

At dinner that night, I picked at my food. Jenny asked if she could be excused. I looked at Sara and then at Jenny.

"Sure, in a minute, but there's something we need to talk about, Jenny," I said to her.

"I'm not in trouble, am I?" she said.

I smiled at her. The innocence of her question really hit me, even though I could have predicted it.

"No," I said with a small laugh, "but your mom and I need to tell you something."

I turned fully to her, scooting my chair and leaning in toward her.

"I was at the doctor today. There is something wrong with my kidney and I'm going to have an operation next week to fix it."

I paused and, as I did so, she studied my face.

"You're not going to die, are you, Dad?" she asked, her almond-shaped eyes wide open. She looked at her mom, seeking reassurance.

"Dad will be okay," Sara said, "but this is a big operation and it will take your dad a while to recover."

Jenny looked back at me and moved toward me. She gave me a hug and held me tight.

"I love you, Dad," she said. She almost immediately added, "You don't have cancer like mom, do you?"

Moment of truth time.

"I have a tumor in my kidney and they are going to take it out. So, yes, I have cancer," I said.

Tears came to her eyes and she began to cry.

"Are you as sick as Mom? Are you really going to be all right?"

"The doctor said he's sure it'll be fine," I said. "We just need to get this taken care of. If we do it quickly, I'll be okay."

She continued to cry. Sara joined us for a group hug. I put my arms around the two of them.

"You remember how sick Mom was? And the doctors were able to make her better. We just need to believe in the doctors and have faith it'll be all right. I believe it will be and I'm the one who has the most to worry about, right?"

Jenny looked into my eyes and asked if I was scared.

"I am a little," I said. "Any time we don't know for certain what will happen, it can be kind of scary. I know Dr. Vora is a very good doctor, and he'll take good care of me."

My words seemed to help her process what she was being told. Her tears stopped and she stepped back.

"If you think it will be okay, then I will too," she said with a bit of resolve in her voice.

"I'll be fine, Jenny," I said. "Why don't you get ready for bed. You have school tomorrow and need your shower."

Sara went upstairs with her, and I was left to my thoughts.

One down. Andrew to go. I had no idea where he was. I figured he was in California, but he could be who knows where on a project for AmeriCorps. In any event, it was always a chore to reach him. We had the office number, but he did not have a cell phone. We had set a schedule with him, having him call in on a regular basis. Fortunately, this was his night to call.

The phone rang around 9:00 p.m. and, after a brief round of small talk, I told him that I had something we needed to discuss. He got quiet as I walked him through the specifics. The concern was obvious in his voice. But the usual Andrew logic kicked in and he asked if he should come home.

"No, I'll be okay," I said. "This is a big surgery, though. They're telling me I'll be off six weeks, recovering. So I probably won't be back at work until after the first of the year."

"How is Mom doing with this?" he asked.

"She has been great, just like you would expect," I said. "She's getting stronger all the time, so she should be able to help me as I recover. Her cancer seems to be in remission right now. It should all be good."

A pause followed before he asked me if I was confident they had the right diagnosis.

I told him that I had confidence in Dr. Vora and that Dr. Decker was comfortable with him as a surgeon. He pressed the issue of coming home, but I told him I wanted him to stay focused on his work for AmeriCorps. Besides, we'd see him at Christmas. He clearly wanted to be kept informed and I promised him we'd keep him in the loop, just as we did with his mom's illness.

"All right," he said. "I love you, Dad."

"I love you, too, Scooze," I said.

I hung up and sighed. The toughest part was over.

A scan and surgery awaited.

I thought about a line from a Tom Petty song that said waiting is the hardest part. How true.

The same lyrics played in my head on Saturday as I headed to the hospital for my MRI. I felt cold and turned up the heat. It reminded me of how cold hospitals always seemed and how cold I'd felt hearing the news about Sara's cancer—every time.

Once at the hospital, I took a quick look at some paper-work, gave the clerk my insurance card, and got into a hospital gown. I was still cold and the hospital gown didn't help. I thought of what was ahead. I wasn't fond of closed-in spaces, and I knew I'd be placed in a tube-like structure for the scan. I had taken a valium on the way to the hospital and was beginning to feel its effects. I knew I would become more relaxed as the drug worked within my system.

When I was finally called, I entered the imaging area and the technician described the procedure. There would be two scans, one without contrast and one with it. I moved to the sliding tray that would serve as my home for most of the next hour. The only question I had for her was whether I could listen to some music.

"Sure," the nurse said. "Did you bring something?"

"Yes," I said, handing her the Tom Petty CD I had brought. It included the song I was humming on the drive to the hospital. "If I could listen to this, it would help."

"No problem," she said with a smile. "Lots of people get claustrophobic in this situation. The music will help. Just take deep breaths and relax. It will be over before you know it.

"We'll be able to hear you throughout the procedure, so if you need something or get to feeling too uncomfortable, let us know. Oh, and it is very important that you remain very still so we get proper images."

I took a deep breath and was rolled into the massive machine. The valium had taken hold and the space was close, but it was not as intimidating as I expected.

Forty-five minutes later, we were done. I was back on the road home by 3:40 a.m., glad to be in my car, where I could crank up the heater. I was still cold.

By 4:15, I was back in bed. I wondered what the images showed but quickly drifted off to sleep. Another step in the journey was complete. I was ever closer to the surgery that would save my life.

The next few days ran together as everything fell into place for my surgery. I spent part of my weekend contacting friends and family, letting them know of my situation.

Sara and I talked after Jenny went to bed on Sunday night, trying to get our bearings on all that was happening.

"My head is still spinning," I admitted. "So much has happened in the past ten days. It's just surreal."

She looked deeply into my eyes and moved closer on the leather loveseat in our family room.

"I know. I feel the same way," she said. She took my right hand in her hands and squeezed it tightly. A period of silence followed as we both let our imaginations roll on.

"What are you feeling right now?" she asked, exhibiting more of her therapist role than I was used to seeing. She peered ever more deeply into my eyes.

"I'm not sure. I don't know how I feel, other than a bit numb," I said. "One thing I do know is that I'm not afraid. Maybe it's because I have had no symptoms. Maybe it's because I've been dealing with mortality through your cancer. I'm not sure. But I am sure I'm not scared."

If Sara was surprised, she didn't show it.

"Our lives have had so many twists and turns, I wonder sometimes if we truly have become numb to it all," she said.

The numbness that I had grown accustomed to with Sara's cancer battle was similar to the feeling I was experiencing. But, then again, it wasn't quite the same. As close as I had been to Sara through the seventeen years since she was first diagnosed, this felt significantly different. I was the patient this time.

"I really trust the doctors and I believe they have all this right," I said. "But there is always that nugget of doubt—that sense they could be wrong."

"There is no benefit in going there," Sara warned. "There is no reason to think anything other than you'll have the surgery, they will get the cancer, everything will go as they have said it will, and our lives will go on."

As usual, her perspective was dead on. Negativity was a drain. I told her I would focus on being positive.

The next morning, I was at my office when my assistant buzzed my office.

"There's a Dr. Vora on the phone for you," she said.

I wondered why he was calling and anxiously punched the button to take his call.

"Hello, Dr. Vora," I said. "I'm looking forward to seeing you Wednesday so we can get this thing over with. I assume you're calling about my MRI. Is everything okay?"

"Yes, Ron, I am calling about the MRI," he said. "The tumor in your left kidney is as I expected. I'm ninety-nine percent certain we'll have to remove your kidney because of the position of the mass. The scan also showed something we didn't expect. There's a small mass in your right kidney. It's very unusual. I'm not sure what it is; we really can't tell. But I wouldn't be doing what is in your best interests if I had you in surgery and didn't investigate this further."

My mind immediately shifted back to the spinning, out of control mode.

"So, what does that mean? Are you saying you'll have to cut me on both sides?" I asked in disbelief.

"Yes, Ron. I'm afraid that *is* what I am saying," he replied. "I really don't like talking about this over the phone, but I wanted to tell you as soon as I had the information."

I quickly slipped back to that moment less than two weeks earlier when Dr. Khilanani reached me by cell phone at the racetrack. All kinds of things flooded my mind, making it difficult to concentrate on what he was saying.

I thought back to what we had discussed the previous week in his office. Dr. Vora had told me I would have an incision about a foot in length on my left side. Now he was adding another cut to the equation. I thought of the guy in the illusionist act who lies in a box on a stage and is "cut in half" as part of a show in Vegas.

"We will see you early Wednesday. Don't worry. We will take care of all this then," he said as he concluded the call.

I wondered if the story could get any more complicated and what kind of surprise call I would get next.

I immediately called Sara and told her what Dr. Vora had just said.

There was a long pause on the phone line as Sara digested what I had said.

"So how did he say they will do this?" she asked.

"They will make an incision on my left side first and close me up when they're done. Then they will turn me, cut into my right side, and do an examination of that kidney. This isn't the way I wanted to start my Monday," I said, trying to lighten the moment.

It was nearly impossible to focus on work over the next two days. I did my best to get through the stacks of material I had on my desk, but the looming surgery consumed me and stole me away as I tried to focus on work.

My parents made the trip to Troy Tuesday afternoon. It was nice to have them at the house. We had arranged for them to be there to help by looking after Jenny and generally helping Sara—and me—over the next several days.

My mind was reeling again as Sara and I went to bed Tuesday night. I had spent much of the day getting things in order. It seemed a negative approach to the pending surgery, but it was a necessity. It occurred to me that we had far less to get arranged than I had hoped for at age forty-eight.

Sara asked if I was okay as she slid across the bed and gave me a hug. I admitted I was still numb. It was an odd experience. My mind was racing, but I was a bit removed from it. It was like watching a film and being the lead player at the same time.

"I know that feeling," she said in response, smiling. "It's very unsettling. I try to stay focused on the things that bring me the most joy: you, the kids, my faith. It distracts me and helps quiet my mind."

I heard what she said. She had enough experience dealing with life-and-death issues that she could do that. Maybe I was too new to this. I had tried those strategies; they had yet to fully work.

I managed to sleep only a couple of hours. The alarm pierced the early morning silence. I hadn't needed it. It was still dark as I showered, and I pressed my left side, wondering what was going on in my body. I took a deep breath and tried to focus. All this was beyond my full comprehension.

Sara and I left the house just as the sun was breaking on the horizon. I knew that my situation had to stir up a complicated gumbo of feelings for her. It was certainly stirring them up in me.

It will be days before I can leave, I thought—down one kidney. More importantly, absent one cancerous tumor.

The hospital was a sleepy place, just coming to life, as we entered the main lobby. The smell of Starbucks drifted through the hallways and pulled at me as I observed the line of people who waited for their coffee and lattes. It was more enticing than usual because I'd been ordered to have nothing to eat or drink after midnight.

We went to the hospital's registration area and I checked in. The friendly woman behind the desk seemed a bit too cheery for 6:30 in the morning.

Once checked in, I changed into a hospital gown. I knew it would be my standard attire for the next week. That was a humbling thought. I tied the gown strings and crawled into bed. The nurse came in with Sara. While Sara held my hand, the nurse went through her litany of questions. I knew it was all necessary, but I just wanted to get on with it. As the nurse was starting my IV, the anesthesiologist came by to introduce himself and confirm my health background. The nurse and anesthesiologist left and I was alone with Sara only briefly before Dr. Vora entered.

He asked if I was ready.

"I am," I said. "The more important question is, are you ready? I'm just going to be hangin' out."

He smiled and told me he was, indeed, ready to go. He went over what would happen in surgery and assured me that he was confident all would go well.

He left and the nurse returned with a little something to help me relax. It began working almost immediately. My cares were drifting away.

An orderly came to wheel me to the surgical suites. I told Sara that I would see her in a few hours. She said she loved me as I was wheeled away.

Lying on the gurney as it rolled down the hall, the lights flashed by and seemed extremely bright as my drug-altered mind tried to hang on to reality. We arrived in the operating room and it was so cold that I started shivering. One of the assisting nurses brought me a blanket, and I heard Dr. Vora's voice somewhere in the room. But the drugs were really kicking in and, honestly, I didn't care. The anesthesiologist leaned in to ask if I was ready to be put under. I said yes.

"Okay," he said. "We'll see you again in a little bit."

When he pushed the plunger on the syringe, I felt a rush in my head and floated away.

The next thing I knew, I was in the ICU where a nurse was standing at my bedside, checking my vital signs. I was groggy and thirsty. She gave me some ice chips, which soothed my parched mouth. My throat hurt and I could barely swallow. The nurse said it was from the tube that had been inserted during the operation.

I was in and out over the next few hours and was happy to see Sara when I next opened my eyes.

"How'd I do?" I asked in a scratchy voice as she leaned in to kiss my forehead.

"You came through with flying colors," she said, smiling and squeezing my hand. "It went like Dr. Vora said it would. They took your left kidney and the tumor. Then they went into your right side to see if they could find anything there. Thankfully, they didn't. Dr. Vora thinks it all went very well."

I dozed in and out for much of the next twenty-four hours. The key to making it work, from a pain perspective, was the epidural that had been placed in my spine. The morphine minimized my pain and pushing the button to activate its delivery became something I learned very quickly.

As is the case with all surgeries today, the doctors want you on your feet within hours after the procedure. I was up that night and walked a short distance down the hall with the assistance of a nurse. It didn't take long, though, for me to want to get back in my bed.

I slowly recovered over the next six days and was finally able to go home. It was great to get back to the house. My mom and dad had been around for the surgery and then went back to their place in Ohio and spent the next few days there before coming back to Troy.

It was two days before Thanksgiving and good to be home for the holiday. I moved very slowly around the house. The epidural was long gone, now replaced by Tylenol 3. After the Thanksgiving weekend, I spent most days at home on my own. Sara was back at work and Jenny back at middle school.

The dogs, Allie and Murphy, were constant companions. Each spent the days lying nearby, keeping an eye on me. It's uncanny how dogs sense when you are in need. Murphy would follow me on my laps from the family room into and through the living room and back through the kitchen to the family room. I would do ten or more laps each day and he was right there with me, following closely behind.

Dr. Vora and I had discussed my recovery schedule, and he recommended I stay home until the first of the year. By the last two weeks in December, I was getting restless. But I abided by his wishes and did not return to work until January.

Through it all, I was growing stronger and was pleased with my progress. I occasionally had that gnawing cancer feeling about what could be lying below the scar on the right side of my abdomen. Both Dr. Vora and the pathologist, who evaluated the tumor they removed, had physically examined my right kidney and found nothing. I was grateful for that.

But I wondered. I wondered why that image in the MRI had caused Dr. Vora to open up my right side, giving me twin twelve-inch scars on my torso. I wanted to believe all was good and would be indefinitely. But my experience with cancer led me to a place that always included doubt. It worried me, but it was generally down on my list of concerns.

Sara and I talked about it one night after I had gone back to work.

"I don't want to believe anything is there," I said as we sat together on the living room loveseat. "But I also wonder what it was that showed up in that scan."

Sara looked at me in the knowing way that she often did when she was preparing to say something poignant.

"You know how this works," she said, matter-of-factly. "There are no guarantees, no certainties. The one thing we have to stay focused on is living our lives a day at a time. We can't jump ahead. But we can't look back, either. We've learned that from my time with cancer. Our lives are great. We have one another. We have Andrew and Jenny. We're blessed to have had great careers and work we enjoy. We have a wonderful home."

She paused for just a moment before adding the pertinent and poignant capstone. "And we are both cancer free."

"I know. We do have a lot to be thankful for," I agreed. "I just get tired of the uncertainty. We never seem to know where this will go. It would be nice to know—even just once."

Sara looked hard into my eyes.

"There are some things we don't know—we won't ever know," she said. "I really believe there are some things we aren't meant to know. Accepting that, living with it, is the only way we can deal with it."

I knew what she said was true. In fact, I had said it to her during one of her "moments" less than a year earlier. Being there for me—being there for each other—had always been one of the strengths of our relationship.

It was her turn to hold me up. As usual, she elevated me by saying the right thing at the right time.

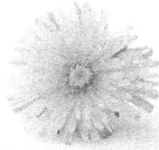

CHAPTER
9

The massive scars on my abdomen were constant reminders of cancer past, as well as the possibility of cancer future. I worked hard to keep it out of my mind and, for the most part, was able to do so.

Sara and I were back at work and things seemed to be on the track we'd been walking down until our cancer-filled 2000 came crashing down on us. As autumn was slipping into early winter, Sara was back at work in the Troy schools as 2000 evolved into 2001.

I was back at work in 2001, too, and disappointed to be watching CART slowly imploding. Bad decision heaped atop bad decision was crushing the racing organization. It was extremely frustrating because we had started to make some progress in bettering the perception of the racing organization. But constant bickering, self-serving decisions, and some bizarre judgments had created a building tsunami that ended up washing CART away. It made going to the office a real challenge most days and diminished my enthusiasm for the work.

We conducted race events in countries around the world, and in September of 2001, I went to Berlin to represent the organization in advance of a race in Germany. I had flown overnight from Detroit to get to Berlin. I checked into a small hotel and wanted to take a brief nap before showering and heading to the evening reception.

As I was dozing, I heard something on the only English language television station—CNN—that caught my attention. I opened my eyes and saw smoke billowing from one of the World Trade Center towers in New York City on the small television screen.

The commentators said they believed a small aircraft had hit the building. As I watched, I found it hard to imagine that a plane could crash into one of the tallest and most formidable buildings in the world on a cloudless, sunny Manhattan day, and I sat up to watch more. In a few minutes, the second plane plowed into the other tower and the world was changed forever.

The tragedy was horrible for the families and friends of the thousands who died. We, the CART community, suffered through the tragedy and experienced our agony and pain from afar. We felt very isolated and alone. We were later told that our contingent of roughly 1,500 was the largest group of Americans outside the US, and our government took great pains to make sure we were kept informed and safe.

Of course, like all members of our group, I wished I was home with my family. But we had a race to conduct.

As the events of September 11 played out, they reached into our family in a way we could not have expected.

We knew when Jenny started middle school in the fall of 2000 that it would be a difficult time for her. Beyond the normal angst that comes with being a kid in the squeeze between elementary and high school, we suspected that changing classes and increased academic pressure would combine with the ever present and sometimes nasty chatter among middle school kids to be a real challenge for her.

Jenny managed to get through sixth grade and for a few days as she started seventh grade in 2001, she did all right before her behavior began to deteriorate. She refused to sit in math class. She would regularly remove herself by saying she had to go to the restroom. She was moody and seemed angry. As the pressure and stress of middle school increased, so did her bizarre behavior. It came to a crescendo when she became agitated, kicked an assistant principal, and was suspended.

Kids who had been removed from school were required to attend classes in a nearby Boys and Girls Club, where they talked with a counselor, did their schoolwork, and tried to work through their behavioral issues. For some reason, Jenny became worked up during her first day in the "suspension school" and dealt with her feelings by using her foot to make her point, kicking a fellow student. The result? Suspension from the suspension school. Her behavior continued to spiral out of control and we, along with the school administration, decided it would be best if she was placed in a school for students with emotional and behavioral issues.

Jenny was slowly starting to adjust to this school and continued her emotional roller coaster until she spiraled out of control on September 11.

The Friday before I left for Europe, I had been in New York on business. I was home on the weekend and then set out for Germany. For some reason, in Jenny's mind I was still in New York City when the September 11 attacks occurred.

The television coverage was on at school. She heard the staff talking about the Twin Towers and the devastation and death. Her thinking put two and two together and she came to the conclusion that I was somehow involved in the tragedy.

As her day edged along, she became more and more agitated. The staff felt it best that Sara pick her up. After Jenny got into the car, Sara drove a short distance onto a main thoroughfare and Jenny opened the door, jumped from the car, and ran into traffic. Sara somehow managed to gather her up and back into the car. But the episode meant we were faced with putting Jenny in a place where she could no longer endanger herself or others.

Sara contacted our therapist and Jenny ended up at Kingswood, a psychiatric facility on notorious Eight Mile Road at the north edge of Detroit. She was there when I returned from our European races and we met with Jenny's psychiatrist. He had thoroughly reviewed Jennys case and had come to a significant conclusion.

"I believe we are at a point where we must comprehensively deal with the issues of Jenny's illness," he said. "This history of stabilizing her and putting her back on the street is not helpful, nor is it working. If we don't deal with this head-on, I think we could lose her. I'm of the opinion that we should keep her here and observe her for more than thirty days, and that will qualify her for Medicaid. Then the cost of the longer-term treatment that she really needs will be covered."

We had a relationship with Easter Seals, the organization Oakland County worked with in managing psychiatric, emotional, and behavioral issues. They considered Jenny's case and immediately began exploring placement options.

She ended up in Children's Home of Detroit, a locked, twenty-four-hour psychiatric unit that sat on the north side of General Motors' huge campus in Warren.

Her placement made Sara and me empty nesters. Andrew was off at Western Michigan University in Kalamazoo. He had completed his AmeriCorps stint in early August and had started his college career. We moved him into his dorm the first of September.

I was slowly putting the mounting misery of work behind me. We grappled with Jenny's absence and struggled to come to grips with the significance of her illness. It felt as if we had lost a piece of her, and we wondered if we would ever get it—and her—back.

Jenny's well-being became the focus of our lives during the final months of 2001. We were in and out of numerous meetings with psychiatrists, psychologists, social workers, doctors, nurses, insurance people, and hospital administrators. The amount of time we devoted to it was massive.

We continued our daily routines as best we could. CART had become a quagmire of strange decisions, and we muddled through to somehow finish our racing season in early November. And, in spite of Jenny's troubles, Sara and I were enjoying the time we had together.

Sara had ongoing tests, scans, and checkups. She also had treatments on a regular basis in the form of preventive drugs administered by infusion. But otherwise, life had returned to normal—at least as normal as it gets when you've had significant bouts with cancer and are always on cancer watch. We joked about, and enjoyed, our "scan dates" on Friday or Saturday nights.

One particular Friday evening, Sara had an evening appointment for a brain scan. The following morning, Sara and I headed to our favorite breakfast place and then off to do some shopping. We were out until later in the afternoon and brought our purchases home, unloaded them, and sat down at the kitchen table to catch our breath. Sara lifted the phone from its wall mount and discovered the quick beeps indicating we had voicemail messages.

She dialed into the system and found one message in the queue. She recognized the voice of the on-call oncologist from Cancer Care, one of Dr. Decker's partners. Sara's face turned serious as she listened.

"Hello, Sara," said the female voice in the recorded message as Sara and I shared the handset to listen. "This is Marianne Huben. I'm calling about your scan last night. I'm sorry to leave a message, but you need to go to the hospital ER as soon as you get this message. The scan showed a tumor in your brain that is in a very sensitive area, and I'm concerned it could cause an issue if not treated immediately. I have left word at the ER in Royal Oak regarding your admission. They will be waiting for you and will get you into a room right away so we can treat this. I don't want to sound dramatic, but I can't overstate the urgency. I encourage you to leave for the hospital after listening to this. Again, I'm sorry to leave this news in a message, but it has the potential to be serious. I'll see you soon."

The reality of cancer—again—had come crashing down on us.

"Well," I said as I looked into Sara's eyes, "it looks like we will have another date night at Beaumont."

She laughed weakly and I was glad I could break the tension with a bit of humor. I knew, though, that was all the further that tact could go. We were faced with what sounded like a very serious situation and had to act promptly. The lightheartedness of our day evaporated with the message.

"Let me get a few things together and then we can go," she said, a note of dejection in her voice as she headed toward the stairs.

I joined her in our bedroom as she took a few minutes to pack a couple of nightgowns, some panties, and a robe, as well as another pair of jeans and a different top.

"I'm ready to go," she said as she walked toward me with a tear trickling down her right cheek. "The next chapter in all this is starting, I guess. We'll keep fighting like always. Let's go."

I held her hand as I led her down the narrow, steep staircase. I had often wondered why the builder designed it that way and thought of how difficult the stairs could be to negotiate, especially for someone with physical challenges. We got in the car and headed to the place that had become our second home. There was an odd sense of comfort as I pulled into the circle that led to the massive doors of the Beaumont Emergency Room.

A security officer met us and helped Sara into a wheelchair. I returned to the car, moved it into the parking lot, and returned to the hospital. I asked for Sara and the admitting nurse said she had already been moved to the ER. The first nurse I saw in the ER pointed me in the right direction and I found Sara already lying on a gurney in a hallway toward the back of the emergency room. All the draped exam areas were occupied so we waited for one of the curtained spaces as a nurse gathered Sara's vital signs.

"They've contacted Dr. Huben and she'll be here soon," Sara said to bring me up-to-speed as the sound of separating Velcro strips on the blood pressure cuff broke through the low-level noise. The nurse took her temperature and placed an oximeter on her left index finger.

A voice drifted over my left shoulder. It was one of the emergency room docs and he was stopping to give us an update.

"Dr. Huben is on her way in," he said, "but in the meantime, we want to begin an IV of steroids. The scan you had last night shows swelling in your brain and the risk of pressure from a tumor in the region near your brain stem. As quickly as we can, we need to begin to bring the swelling down to minimize the potential for anything to occur."

He asked Sara several questions and initiated a brief neurological exam, checking her ability to squeeze his fingers and making certain the sense of feeling was normal in her fingers and toes. He touched her face to make certain she had no numbness and ran his small metal hammer's handle into the sensitive areas of her feet, legs, hands, and arms. All came back normal.

A nurse attached an IV bag using Sara's chest port.

"I think we are good to go. Just relax and when Dr. Huben arrives, we'll send her back to you," the nurse said. "I'm sorry we've had to place you here right now. Full up," she added, with a little laugh. "They're working to get you a room, and I think we'll be able to do that soon. Let's hope that happens before long."

The nurse returned with a volunteer who pushed the bed out of the ER to begin the journey to Sara's room. I noticed that the massive hospital was strangely quiet as she transported Sara to Beaumont's seventh floor cancer unit. Not long after Sara was carefully situated into the bed nearest the door, Dr. Huben stuck her head into the room.

She apologized for leaving the message as she did and reiterated that she had only done so because she needed to get Sara to the hospital as quickly as possible.

Sara assured her it was fine. She had developed a good relationship with Dr. Huben over the past few years and was very comfortable with her.

"I really don't have any pain or other symptoms," Sara said. "I guess I should be really happy we did the scan. But I feel fine."

Dr. Huben leaned into the edge of Sara's hospital bed to start a brief exam as she explained the details.

"The scan was very clear. There are four tumors in your brain. One is very near your brain stem. You know anatomy well enough to understand that is a very sensitive part of the brain. It controls critical autonomic functions: breathing, sight, swallowing."

I could see in Sara's eyes that she fully understood and was surprised to hear her offer a lighthearted response.

"You sound so serious, Marianne," Sara said, chiding Dr. Huben as the corners of her mouth rose into a small smile as she tried to lighten the moment. "I'm just glad we found this. We now know what we are up against. I have suspected for a while this could happen."

Dr. Huben seemed relieved at Sara's response. She concluded her exam and was putting her instruments back in her bag as she spoke.

"We'll continue with the steroids until we think it's safe to take you off them. Then we'll watch you for a day or two to make sure the swelling doesn't return. I think the steroids will be all we need to bring this under control. But it was extremely important that you got here to start treatment. I didn't want to run the risk of your having a vital function going awry."

I looked across the bed and into Marianne's eyes. She knew what I was going to ask.

"So where do we go from here?" I asked. "What are the longer-term options?"

She didn't hesitate. She said radiation was the standard of care for a situation like this. Surgery would be a consideration. She also said there were new treatments using lasers that we would need to look into. That pretty much summed up the options. The body has a natural line of defense that fastidiously protects the head from the vast majority of chemo drugs, and science had not yet figured out a way to circumvent that system.

Sara looked at me and, seeing that I was satisfied with Dr. Huben's response, turned back to her.

"I know we'll look into all the options and, as always, my job is to be the best patient I can be," she said. "I'm sure we'll get it figured out."

I could see Marianne relax a bit with Sara's words.

"You are always such a wonderful patient, Sara, and you provide us insights that are very useful as we treat you," the doctor said. "You're right. We *will* figure it out."

Dr. Huben turned toward the door, told us she would return in the morning, and said good night.

The gravity of the situation settled over me like a heavy cloud. Just a few hours earlier, we had been at Hudson's, beginning our Christmas shopping. Being normal. It now felt like that was days ago. The cancer we so abhorred had dropped straight back into the center of our lives, commanding our attention. It was about 9:00 p.m. when Sara caught me nodding off. She reached down from her bed and shook my knee as the television droned on in the background.

"You need to go home and get some sleep," she said. "And the dogs need you. They get lonely when we leave them for so long. Plus, I don't want you to have to clean up after them."

I rose from the chair and stared at the little television, trying to get my focus.

I leaned in to give her a kiss and she hugged me and held on longer than usual.

"I love you so very much," she said. "You know we'll beat this thing. We just need to get a plan and make it happen."

"I know," I responded. "We'll push it back. I have to say, it was great to have a break from it. I was just beginning to enjoy our time away from this stuff. But it will be okay."

I kissed her, told her I loved her, and left. My mind was unsettled on the drive home. A new normal had yet again come to be. I took stock of all the changes that had and were occurring. Sara's cancer was back and it had returned with a vengeance. The metastasis had gone from her liver to her brain. Serious stuff.

I recalled our days in college at Colorado State. More than once, when she had a headache, Sara half-jokingly wondered about having a brain tumor. It really hit me and I pondered the newest cancer battle we faced. The power of suggestion, of creating your reality, popped into my mind but I dismissed it, knowing it served no real benefit.

It was critical that we do all we could to mitigate the impact of these newly discovered tumors. The whirlwind of a cancer-plagued life was gaining momentum again. I knew the feeling and I didn't like where I knew things were going.

Then there was the situation with Jenny. She'd ended up in long-term psychiatric care after spiraling out of control. Fortunately, it seemed we had finally gotten her properly diagnosed. We owed a great deal to the doctor who got her into extended care. She was firmly ensconced at the Children's Home of Detroit and, seemingly, getting under control.

For the boys in the family, change was occurring at a quickening rate. Within the past few months, Andrew had returned from AmeriCorps, started college, and was settling into his college schedule. He seemed pleased with his school and surroundings. As for me, the situation at work had deteriorated to the point that I knew, deep down, I was going to have to leave. And I was ready to do so. CART was self-destructing and those of us on the inside could do little to slow its demise.

It was liberating to know that I would probably soon be moving on. Doing PR for an organization bent on destroying itself is miserable. I had begun to investigate opportunities but was hamstrung in searching because of Sara's and Jenny's situations.

We had always been willing to embrace change. It was reflected in our career choices and our willingness to seek new opportunities and adventures. It was becoming clear, though, that now was not the time. We needed stability. Sara needed to know that we would focus on the latest battle in her never-ending war against cancer and not have the distractions of moving and starting a new life in some other city. The next morning, I found Sara sitting up in her bed, smiling at me as I entered her room, and leaned in to kiss her and give her a hug.

"I'm so glad you're here," she said. "It's been a tough few hours. The woman in the bed next to me died during the night."

She paused and looked away, and I knew she was fighting off tears. When she turned back, she looked into my eyes.

"I don't want that to ever be me—to die in the hospital. They are so good to us as patients and work so hard to try to save us. But they don't deal with dying very well. The way they handled it in the middle of the night felt cold."

I sensed another pivotal moment in our cancer journey was unfolding, and I listened to Sara intently.

"So, what are you saying?" I asked.

"I think I would like to explore where it would be best to do hospice care," she said. "When things settle down and I am able to get back out and do things, I want to be able to get around and check out different places. I don't know anything about it, really. But I do know hospice has a very different approach to this kind of thing, and it is more sensitive to dealing with dying."

I thought hard about what she had just said. This was a conversation that most couples in their forties probably weren't having on a Sunday morning. But it was important, particularly for Sara, and I made sure I didn't dismiss it.

"I can start to gather a few things about it and check around if you want," I said.

"I think it's something I want to do on my own," she replied. "It'll give me something to do. I need some things to focus on since I probably won't be returning to work. I'll do my research and then bring you into it when I have found places I like."

It was a plan and I understood it was important to step aside and let her run with this.

"Okay, just let me know when you want me to get involved."

I settled into the chair that now sat between the two beds. The curtain between the beds was pulled back and I looked out the window. The previous night the curtain had been closed and a waning life had filled the space on the window side of the divider. How quickly the world changes, I thought.

And now, our world had, yet again, reset to a new normal. I had to accept the change. Sara was acknowledging her mortality, something we had never actually addressed.

Sara spent the next couple of days in the hospital. Drs. Huben and Decker each came by and voiced how pleased they were with the progress she was making. The tumors in her brain were responding to the intense IV treatments. As the swelling diminished, the pressure in her brain lessened, minimizing the potential for something negative to occur.

A radiation oncologist came by and talked with Sara about beginning treatments. She recalled how she had gone through radiation treatments when she had her recurrence in 1989. The side effects generally are relatively minor with radiation. There is some soreness and redness in the treated area and a general feeling of tiredness. Otherwise, it goes as smoothly as something like that can.

Sara's treatments'began the following week, and she was scheduled at the same time each weekday morning. She was to have twenty treatments in total.

I took her to the Beaumont Radiology area for the first one. It was the first time I had gone through this particular form of treatment with her. When she had her radiation in Denver, I had moved ahead to Milwaukee, starting my new job. I reminded her of that and said I was sorry I was not around for her then. She smiled and told me that she was just happy I was able to be with her now.

One of the things that is both good and bad about radiation treatment is that you can only safely have a specific number of treatments before the physicians say, "No more," for that particular area. Sara had reached that amount of radiation in her chest, but she could have the treatments that were about to occur on her head without any issues.

A technician appeared and asked Sara if she was ready for her treatment. I thought how much fun it would be to say, just once, "No, I'm not ready. Let's wait for a couple hours." It was a little silly, but underlying it was the constant feeling of having no control that accompanies dealing with cancer. To manage a little piece of it occasionally would provide a miniscule feeling of triumph against the disease and all that goes with it.

Sara went in for her treatment and returned forty-five minutes later. I asked how it had gone.

"Well, the people are very nice and they were very helpful," she said. "It's easy for me. All I had to do was lie down and stay still.

"I had to laugh as they finished the prep for my treatment," she continued. "It really gets me that this is supposed to be making you better and, after they get you situated, they almost run out of the room, close the massive doors, peer in at you through little windows, and talk to you on a microphone system. It seems totally counter to why you are here. You wonder how it can make you better when they avoid it at all costs."

I laughed at the mental picture I had of it, an exaggeration of what Sara said. I envisioned people walking slowly around the room in 1950s science fiction movie space suits. Sara was so right about it. The bottom line, though, was that this radiation thing, like all her treatments, was deadly serious.

Her treatments continued through the beginning of the year, and a scan at their conclusion confirmed the tumors had stabilized and did not appear to be growing.

Sara's checkups and infusion treatments continued. While the Taxol treatments were behind her, each month she received an infusion of Zometa, a drug designed to manage metastases in bone. Sara's countless scans had shown small spots of cancer in some of her bones, particularly in her lower back and spine, so Dr. Decker had prescribed the drug to minimize the impact. With the metastases in her liver and brain, we pretty much placed the cancer in her bones on the back burner. Fortunately, Sara had no bone pain with the disease but had agreed to continue the treatments.

Sara also had occasional infusions of Procrit, a drug that helps bolster red blood cell counts to avoid anemia. She regularly received the drug when she was in the throes of Taxol chemotherapy to help her maintain her red blood count. The need for that had diminished as she moved further from the chemo treatments but, with the radiation, there was a need to revisit use of the drug.

As Sara was further evaluated, Dr. Decker and his team determined that it was possible to do surgery to remove the tumors from her brain. Sara was referred to a neurologist and surgeon at Beaumont. However, after reviewing all the scans and Sara's history, it was decided that, since the tumors were as small as they were, there was potential to do damage to adjacent tissue that could affect her autonomic functions. The greatest concern was for the tumor located near her brain stem. Because of its relatively small size, the surgeon was very concerned about tissue damage and risks associated with that if they performed surgery.

While surgery was ruled out as 2002 unfolded, there were other options. Dr. Decker recommended a chemo treatment that had shown some promise for breast cancer patients with brain metastases. The problem was that, most of the time, the treatment worked in a limited way. While a terrific filter in most cases, the blood-brain barrier creates a problem when trying to treat cancer that has traveled to the brain. Even so, Sara took the treatment as part of her infusion.

Winter was winding down and we made one of the more than four hundred trips to Beaumont we would make during Sara's illness. This trip was to discuss our options with Dr. Decker. They included surgery, though this was not a good option. They also included continuing chemotherapy, which Sara was doing, but which, at best, was marginally effective. We could also do nothing, a scenario with which we were not comfortable. Or she could have a stereotactic procedure that would use very focused, laser-like beams of intense light to essentially neutralize the tumors.

After considering the choices, we agreed we would investigate the stereotactic procedure. It seemed to offer a decent upside and it was noninvasive—something very important to us because it allowed Sara to maintain her reasonably good quality of life.

Unbeknown to us, a generous gift was in the offing that would allow us to spend time together in a way we never expected.

CHAPTER
10

I had vacated my position at CART, so I had all the time I needed to be with Sara. While the CART situation had been stressful and something I had looked forward to ending, the way it finally came down was surprising.

CART had fired its CEO in the early fall and brought in Christopher Pook to manage the organization. Chris was known as a sometimes ruthless but brilliant and successful negotiator and manager. He was also rumored to be not very friendly to staff. One day in December, Chris and I arrived at work at the same time and made small talk as we walked in together.

I had been wondering how he would handle my presence in the organization. He had brought in another communications and PR guy when he arrived, someone with whom he had worked for years. I suspected my days were numbered. But as is so often the case in corporate life, no real plan had been laid out for the transition—at least for me.

As the elevator arrived at our floor, he asked me to come by his office after I got situated. Here we go, I thought. He was going to show his true colors and let me go before Christmas, a pretty coldhearted thing, but about what I expected. I placed my briefcase in my office, got a cup of coffee, and walked toward the other end of the floor where Chris' office occupied the northeast corner.

"Thanks for coming by, Ron," Chris said when I was shown in. He moved toward the large black leather sofa in his office and motioned for me to sit. I did, and he joined me, sitting on the opposite end of the couch.

"We've been through a lot and seen a lot of changes since we first met in 1982," he said. I was surprised he remembered me from my Sports Car Club of America days, nearly two decades earlier, when he was head of the Grand Prix and Formula One race in Long Beach, California, and I was working for the Sports Car Club of America.

"Yes," I said. "A lot has gone on since then. Long Beach was a much different place then. I remember seedy tattoo parlors adjacent to the course, a line of dumpy bars, and the flashing lights of a porn theater on the front straightaway across from the pit lane. Not exactly like Monte Carlo."

Chris laughed. My comment put us both a bit more at ease.

"Yes, it was a lot different place in 1982," he said. "It's a great testament to what a major event can do to help build a city. I'm proud of what we have done there."

He paused to allow for a transition to the subject of our meeting and then continued.

"I suspect you know why I asked you to come by. The organization is changing, Ron, and you know we are heading in a different direction. That includes what we are going to do with the communications function."

I looked directly into his eyes as he spoke. He didn't blink, but did look down a bit at the black leather sofa.

"I understand, Chris," I said. "You know, it seems like a very long time ago that I came to CART, and I'm ready to move on and do something else. Of course, with Sara's illness being the top priority in my life, I'm not sure what I'll do. But even if things were the same here, it would be extremely difficult for me to continue. I need to be with her and the travel with this job is killer, as you know."

Chris looked hard at me and his face softened.

"I can't imagine what you're going through with Sara's cancer," he said. "And I know of your daughter's challenges, too. You have my deepest sympathy. I also know it's been a very difficult time to try to place CART in a positive light with all that has gone on here, and I want you to know that both the board and I truly appreciate all you have done."

I thanked him for the recognition.

"As we talked about your circumstances, we wanted to make sure you're able to be with Sara as you need to be," he said, building toward the bottom line of the discussion. He paused for what seemed a long time before continuing.

"On behalf of the board, I'm offering you your full salary and benefits for all of 2002."

I was stunned. Had I heard right? I had been with the company since the end of 1996, but never expected as generous an exit package as this. This would, as I readily knew, cost them more than $200,000. I immediately thought of how I had to fight tooth and nail to get a few thousand dollars for any number of PR programs and wondered how difficult it had been to get this done. Chris's words caused me to tear up, and I stared away from him and out the corner office windows.

"Chris, I don't know what to say. This is wonderful," I said, a big smile breaking across my face. "I could never have expected this. It's very generous, and I am extremely grateful."

Chris smiled and stood. It was obvious he was genuinely touched that he had been able to make this offer. He came toward me to shake my hand and offered one last comment.

"This is the retirement you and Sara will never have. Enjoy your time together—and don't worry about this place. We may ask for your help on a couple of projects, but don't expect us to bother you much. This is your time."

We shook hands and he continued toward me, embracing me and patting my back as we briefly hugged. Like mine, his eyes were moist.

When he stepped back, he told me to have a wonderful holiday. So much for the ruthlessness of Chris Pook.

It was as if a huge weight had been lifted from me. I could now spend the time I wanted with Sara and not have to worry about how I was going to pay the mortgage and all our bills. It was almost too good to be true.

I called Sara to explain what had just happened. There was a long pause and I could hear her trying to stifle her crying before she finally spoke.

"We live with the adversity we have in our lives every day and sometimes it causes us to get bogged down in that reality," she said. "It's easy to lose sight of the fact that there is a lot of good out there. This proves we can never lose sight of that."

She was so right.

"I'm so excited about this. I never thought I'd say that about losing my job," I said, enthusiasm in my voice. "Let's sit down tonight and begin to plan how we can spend our time over the next year. I can't wait to be able to be with you every day so we can relax and enjoy being together."

With Andrew at school and Jenny at the Children's Home of Detroit, we were free to do things we wanted to do—travel, see friends and family—as much as Sara was able.

It was not foreign to us to be off together although it seemed like a long time since we had been able to do so. We had done long weekend getaways when we lived in Wisconsin, with my parents watching the kids as we traveled.

Those trips, though, had always been compacted by our need to return to work. Now we would be able to spend time traveling in a more relaxed manner. We mapped out a plan that included a "Lap of Lake Michigan" driving tour as well as a trip to Colorado to visit friends and Sara's family. We considered some other options, but those two were definite excursions we placed on our calendar.

It was great to have things to look forward to—something often lacking in our recent existence, and the enthusiasm for our trip schedule helped carry us for the next few months. We joked about making sure it was not perceived as "The Sara Richards Farewell Tour." While we realized there was some truth to that notion, we chose to stay focused on how this would be a great chance to get away and see people we had not been with for a while.

Before we would be able to hit the road, though, we had a couple of matters to address. Sara had to conclude her radiation treatments and regain her strength and energy. And we had to decide about the option of stereotactic surgery.

Early in 2002, we had met with the physician who led that Beaumont program. He started the conversation by verbally reviewing Sara's case. It was obvious he had spent a good deal of time with Dr. Decker and Sara's ever growing mountain of medical charts and files.

Sara and I listened intently as he laid out the "surgery." Essentially, it seemed no different than the radiation she had just concluded. There appeared to be no potential issues with its application. But there was a nagging concern. Could he assure us there would be no harm to tissue adjacent to the tumors? That was a critical part of this option, and we were hopeful but cautious.

Sara's list of questions placed that at the top. She had done her homework and developed a comprehensive list of questions, most dealing with the executional aspects of the surgery.

The doctor looked intently across his desk, first at Sara and then me. He smiled, then spoke.

"Sara, first off, I want to tell you how much I'm awed by what you have endured. You deserve a lot of credit. Understand that this is a surgical procedure. It has been proven to be safe and it's noninvasive. Can I absolutely guarantee there will be no collateral tissue damage? I cannot. But I'm extremely confident this can be done with no resulting issues. Like any procedure, there are risks. I wouldn't be honest if I said those risks were minimal. They're not. That said, I'm convinced that this procedure will improve your situation."

We didn't have to decide at that moment, but we had spent a good amount of time discussing it prior to the meeting and decided we would proceed if we were comfortable with this doctor and his explanation. We were, and Sara spoke.

"This is something I'm pretty certain I want to do. I understand there are risks, but there is a greater risk in not doing anything. I'd like to move forward and do this."

The smile returned to his face.

"Great," he said. "Then let's get started."

Getting on the schedule was the next hurdle. It was amazing just how much time these massive and expensive machines were in use. It was rare that someone wasn't being zapped with radiation.

We experienced that, firsthand, the day of the procedure.

It was early in the spring and we arrived at Beaumont around 7:30 a.m. The procedure itself wouldn't last very long, but the prep was excruciatingly slow and time consuming. As the day progressed, we realized we were in for a much longer stay than we anticipated.

Sara had gowned up and was ready for the next step, which, both of us knew, was the most difficult part of the day. A large, metal halo was to go around her head. It was secured to a smaller circle that sat upon her head. That halo was to be attached to her skull with four screws—two into her forehead and the other two into the back of her head.

The technician came and took Sara away for this piece of the process. She returned to the waiting area about forty-five minutes later, the halo firmly attached to her skull. We dabbed her forehead below the marks the screws had made as blood oozed from the wounds. Sara's sister, Cyndi, had come to Royal Oak to be with us through the day and her presence helped pass the time as we waited . . . and waited . . . and waited.

Finally, as darkness was setting in, a nurse came by and gathered us up. They carefully placed Sara in a wheelchair. Her patience had reached its end and her head and neck were fully feeling the weight of the halo. She looked at Cyndi and I and said how much she appreciated us spending our day with her and how she was sorry it had taken so long.

We followed Sara and the nurse to the waiting area, and the doctor appeared almost immediately. He smiled and apologized for the long wait. He asked if I would like to come into the control area so he could share what he and his team would be doing. I was happy to have the opportunity and followed him into a darkened room that featured a window into the space where they were preparing Sara. I watched as they literally locked her head into place to ensure the intense beams of light would engage only the tumors.

Sara's physician directed me to sit down at the panel of monitors and I did, marveling at the technology that would, hopefully, improve Sara's quality of life while extending her remaining time.

"Ron, here is the scan we took earlier today of Sara's head and brain," he said. "There has been almost no change since the last one a few weeks ago, which is a good thing. The radiation treatments seem to have worked."

He moved closer to the monitor and used his pen to point to the tumors in Sara's brain.

"This tumor, as well as these two, is in a place where we are fully confident we can radiate them to the point that they will no longer be an issue. This tumor, however, is in a very difficult position. And because of that, I'm not comfortable using the same level of energy in our attempt to neutralize it.

It is very near her brain stem. Collateral tissue damage is a possibility and could be a problem."

He paused and I could tell he was choosing his words carefully.

"The reality is that I think we can safely go about seventy-five percent of the intensity that we are using on the other tumors. I wish we could do more, but I don't want the procedure to do any harm. We can hope it will be enough to do the job, but we'll just have to wait and see."

I continued peering at the tumors and wished I could reach into the screen and pull them from her brain.

"I understand," I said, nodding to him. "While I was hopeful we could do the same to each of the tumors, as you said, we certainly don't want Sara's functions to be compromised. We want to improve Sara's quality of life, not jeopardize it. I know you will do the best you can and we trust you. Thank you for being so honest and open. I appreciate your detailed explanation of what you'll be doing."

He nodded but said nothing. I could see in his face that he was frustrated by the information he had just delivered.

I pushed back from the control panel, rose from the chair, and headed to the waiting room. I shared the information with Cyndi and we sat down to wait for the outcome. The procedure began and about a half hour passed before the doctor came into the waiting area.

"It all went as expected," he said, a sense of relief in his voice. "We got the three tumors as I told you we would. We did as we discussed with the fourth and will have to wait and see."

He turned as his nurse assistant came through the door with a clipboard of papers we had to sign in advance of Sara's discharge. The technicians had reentered the room where Sara had been literally bolted to the table. They removed the bolts that had kept her head in place and were taking the halo off her skull.

A few minutes later, she emerged in a wheelchair, small bandages on each of the spots on her forehead and back of her head where, a few minutes before, screws had held the halo in place.

"Well, that was quite a day, wasn't it?" she said with a weak smile. The events of the day were clearly present on her face, and it was obvious she was worn out. "I'm just relieved this is over."

She thanked her sister for being there and said she was *really* ready to go home. We had been at the hospital for nearly twelve hours. We were *all* ready to go home.

Later, Sara and I sat together and talked. I was trying to gauge if it was the right time to tell her about the reduced level of radiation on the fourth tumor. I always tried to err on the side of being transparent, not waiting to talk about what could be a difficult discussion. I decided it was something we should discuss.

I told her what the doctor had said to me in the control room.

"You know," she replied, "I suspected that could be the way this would work out and I'm okay with it. Unfortunately, there is no magic pill that cures this. We've done all we can and I feel good about that. We'll have to see what happens. Maybe it was enough to affect that tumor, too."

It always amazed me that she could look at her situation with such a rational and positive point of view. I wanted to say something, but was at a loss. I, too, was worn out.

We decided it was time for bed. I helped her into her nightgown and waited in the bathroom doorway for her to brush her teeth. As I watched, I thought of her perseverance and toughness. I wondered how I would be reacting to this if I were the patient. She finished brushing her teeth, wiped her face, and looked at me through tired eyes in the large mirror that covered the wall in the small bathroom.

"How are you doing? Are you okay?" she asked, turning and putting her arms around me. "I often wonder that. I'm sorry you have to go through all this. You're such a wonderful husband. It means more to me than you can ever imagine. Fifty years old and we're dealing with all this. Who would have thought it? You know, I often consider all those great days we had in high school and college and think of how we talked of our future. This wasn't part of it."

I hugged her closely and told her I loved her. I didn't say anything more as I steered her to bed. I had folded back the comforter and sheets and helped her to get situated, pulling the covers up to her chin. She offered a tired smile and puckered her lips, luring me in to give her a kiss.

"I love you so much," she said. "You are the best man in the world. You take such good care of me."

I gave her a quick kiss and stared back into her eyes.

"I can't do it any other way," I said. "We've always been here for each other and that will never change."

Her eyes fluttered closed as I pulled back.

I headed downstairs to the kitchen to make a sandwich and spend some time with the dogs before coming back to bed. I called Andrew to let him know the procedure had gone well and as expected. I could hear commotion in the background and thought of how I was intruding on his Saturday night and what Sara and I had just discussed. It was not something that a college kid should have to deal with as he was spending time with his friends. That said, he sounded relieved.

I turned my attention to the dogs as I flipped on the television and took a look at CNN and ESPN. The three of us sat together, me looking toward the television and them staring at me in hopes of getting a scrap of my sandwich. It occurred to me how they needed me, too. It was such a comfort to have them sitting at my side, even if they were focused on my simple dinner. My mind went to how much everyone relied on me in our family. This was far more than the pressure of being a financial provider and normal husband, I thought. The pressure, at times, became almost unbearable. Somehow, some way, though, I seemed to manage.

After a few minutes, I gave the dogs each a piece of my sandwich and the three of us went upstairs and found Sara soundly sleeping. The dogs snuggled into their spots on the floor and me into my side of the bed.

I stared at the darkened ceiling and wondered how long we had before this got *really* serious. It seemed so long ago that we had dealt with that first tumor in Sara's breast. In fact, it had been twenty years. It seemed more than that. I thought of how fortunate we were to have had so many good years together. It didn't, though, diminish my curiosity about the future.

One thing that was certain: as always, there would be another chapter.

It would have been nice, though, if we could have written it.

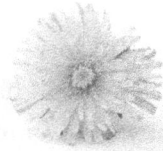

CHAPTER

11

Time passed quickly over the next few weeks and spring-time came into full bloom in southeast Michigan. As always, Jenny was a major focus. Her therapists at the Children's Home of Detroit were cautiously optimistic about her progress. It was slow going, though, and Jenny's oppositional behavior and inability to control her responses to events in her world meant she would be at the psychiatric facility for several more months.

We would usually visit her a couple of times a week. While not necessarily a fair portrayal of CHD, I sometimes thought of scenes from *One Flew Over the Cuckoo's Nest* as we sat with her for an hour in the cafeteria area. Sara would usually bring a game for us to play with Jenny, often a card game, like Uno.

When we visited, Jenny seemed happy to see us at first. Then her mood generally would change and her agitation and anger would rise—usually, for no good reason. Sara was so good with her. Her thousands of hours with adolescent psychiatric patients had given her a great capacity to deal with Jenny.

There often were two or three other families visiting their children when we were there. The most striking characteristic was the tired look in their eyes and the aura of discouragement hanging over them. Completely understandable. But Sara and I worked hard to be positive and upbeat when we were at the home.

By the end of a visit, Jenny often returned from her agitated state and, many times, tears formed in her eyes as she realized we were about to leave. It was no easier for us to leave her than for her to see us go, and we were often quiet on the drive home.

About once a month, Jenny would be allowed to come home on the weekend and, as time passed, she was granted overnight privileges. Those visits were almost always a roller-coaster ride that closely reflected Jenny's mood swings. It wasn't unusual to have an episode requiring physical restraint, nor was it rare for us to take Jenny back to CHD early.

It was difficult to see our daughter at such a place in her life. A genuine sense of sadness hit me when I watched Jenny with Murphy. The little shih tzu had joined our family when Sara, in her never-ending quest to provide Jenny with learning opportunities, decided getting her a dog would help her begin to understand responsibility. Jenny was ten when the Murph joined the household. She truly loved him and loved being with him. But there were a few times during her pre-CHD days when she treated him in a way that left him reluctant to spend time with her. It was sad to watch her try to get him to come and see the look of apprehension on his little face as the scenario played out. She would often just grab him, which seemed to scare him even more.

Then, there was the first time she had come home for a visit after being admitted. It was a warm fall day and she had spent time in her room with her dolls and stuffed animals. Our time was clearly defined and we were in the final hour of her visit. She came downstairs and asked if she could ride her bike. She told me how much she missed it. I said sure and helped her get her bike out of the garage.

It was obvious she saw it as a symbol of freedom and, as I helped her place the purple helmet on her head, tears came to my eyes. I thought back to my days as a kid and how much I loved being on my bike. It was a conveyance that literally, and figuratively, took me away. The wind in your face, the warmth of the sun, the ability to get off on your own—no wonder it was something that was so special for her.

Jenny's plight weighed heavily on us. We wondered if we could have done something differently. We questioned her placement at the Children's Home and if it was really serving to improve her ability to deal with life. The staff seemed good and the Easter Seals agency was convinced this was the best track for Jenny. Of course, we believed we were doing the right thing.

But Sara voiced a sense of guilt, at times, about adopting her. It was especially so as we moved down the path of her illness. We truly loved her and wanted the best for her. We often reinforced to one another how, had Andrew been afflicted with bipolar disorder, we would have done all we could to help him. It was no different with Jenny.

We talked a few times about the fact that if Sara died, I would be raising Jenny on my own. With both of us helping one another as we struggled to manage Jenny and her illness, it was difficult enough. The thought of being a single parent and dealing with her solo was something I chose to push to the corners of my mind. I'd cross that bridge if and when I came to it.

Sara felt well enough many days that we were able to get out to do things we enjoyed: visiting with friends and family; shopping; attending occasional sports, music, or arts events; and a favorite pastime, going to lunch or dinner. They were great diversions from the illness that was now an everyday reality in our lives.

For me, CART's generosity gave us some financial freedom and provided relief from working in a pretty toxic environment. We mapped out the two trips we'd talked about taking. Each would be a week-long trip, the first in May when we flew off to see friends and be with Sara's brother and sister. The second, a car trip, would come in late summer. That excursion would give us the opportunity to see parts of Michigan we had not experienced and connect with a few friends we had not engaged for a while. We were looking forward to getting away for each.

Sara's cancer, and the treatments she endured, had stolen much of her energy. The intense chemo treatments and extensive radiation had sapped her of a good amount of her strength, and, we were discovering, it was gone forever. Like anyone with a severe and chronic illness, she had good days and bad days.

On our trip to Colorado, we first headed to Longmont, north of Denver, to visit with two wonderful friends Tim and Lynn Simmons. It was such a relaxing visit. Their home sits just east of the Rockies and directly below Long's Peak, a 14,000-plus-foot mountain that towers above the Front Range northwest of Denver.

I had gotten to know Tim and Lynn when I was in college, working for Tim as a student in the sports information office at Colorado State University. Tim became a great friend and confidant and, to this day, remains one of the most admired and influential individuals I have in my life.

After dinner, we watched the final shards of light disappear behind the magnificence of the mountains from the cozy patio. We gathered around the warmth of the fire pit to talk, enjoy a beverage, and roast marshmallows.

"I don't know how you've done it," Tim said to Sara and me as we chatted about our journey since Sara's cancer had metastasized. "I really admire how you've managed it all."

Sara and I had grown used to this discussion. We spoke matter-of-factly and from our hearts when we were engaged about it. We embraced the opportunity to convey our belief that, even when faced with adversity, you must stay positive and create a life that is filled with fun, adventure, and satisfaction.

"You know, Tim, everybody has challenges," Sara said after a long pause in the conversation. "Ours just happen to be a little greater than some."

The fire crackled and popped as the flame jumped a bit and spit some sparks at us. Tim thought a moment and responded.

"You guys have had so much on your plate, though. Your cancer, Ron's cancer, Jenny . . . I just don't know how you do it."

I'd been listening quietly, but jumped into the conversation.

"There isn't much you can do about the kinds of things we've gone through," I said. "It's the old adage about how each of us is dealt a hand of cards in life. It's really true that how you play them determines so much about you and the kind of life you end up having. We really believe that. We just try to play the cards we've been dealt in the best way we can."

"There is so much negativity around us every day," Sara added. "It's easy to get bogged down in it, and many people seem to. Each of us has only so much energy and I have less now than I've ever had before. You have to choose how to spend it. Expending your energy on things that are negative has no benefit and only drags you down. I've found that being positive is so much more productive. Your mood is better and, I really believe, it helps you, health-wise."

It was a story we had told over and over, and we would continue to do so. Sara and I had discussed how people seemed to want to learn from us, to get a sense of how, despite all we had endured, we were able to carry on. For us, it was the only way we believed we should handle it.

Sara's "being the best patient I can be" approach expanded beyond her almost constant encounters with the healthcare system. Others had always been drawn to Sara and admired her. She now used that attraction to help people understand how they could achieve a higher plane in their lives, even when faced with difficulties and adversity. Never pushy but always firm, Sara's message seemed to resonate strongly with those who came in contact with her.

For me, it was a bit different. My innate curiosity, a slight bent toward sarcasm, and my education as a journalist and PR professional had shaped me to be more cynical and skeptical. It was difficult to let go of that. Sara and I often discussed our differing perspectives and how she perceived my thinking to be negative. I always disagreed, saying I was a realist, someone who saw a situation for what it was, accepted it, and then worked from a worst-case scenario approach to devise a solution. Then, when things worked out better than anticipated, as they usually did, I was fully prepared to handle it.

Beyond that, people often asked me, point-blank, how I was managing it all. How I was holding up. I generally responded somewhat naïvely, "What else should I do?" Doing what I was doing was the right thing to do. Sure, I knew there were others who might do it differently—become depressed, use drugs and alcohol to cope, maybe have an affair, or even get a divorce. Perhaps it was corny, but I took the wedding vows we had spoken in 1975, seriously. The "in sickness and in health" thing meant something to me. It always would.

The reaction of people was interesting to see. I occasionally sensed that some thought it was a façade, that I really didn't want to be doing what I was doing. In one way, that was true. I had days I wished I wasn't Sara's primary caregiver, that we did not have to endure all that we had. But it had nothing to do with not being there for her. I would never waver. I wished we never had the cancer to deal with in the first place, but I treated my end of it almost as a badge of honor. Doing anything but being there for Sara had never crossed my mind. And I knew she would have done the same for me if the situation was reversed. In fact, she had, during my own encounter with cancer.

Our time in Colorado then took us to visit friends in Golden. We had known Steve and Laurel Saunders for many years after meeting when I worked with Steve at Coors. We had a terrific evening together, catching up, recounting memories, and sharing laughter again and again.

The next day, our tour led us out of the Denver area. We headed to the mountains, driving southwest along US 285, a route we had followed dozens of times when we lived in the state. We drove for a little more than two hours before arriving at the Jump Steady Lodge, near Buena Vista. It was a rustic place, sitting on idyllic Cottonwood Creek. The attraction, other than the towering mountains of the Collegiate Range, were the hot springs that naturally bubbled up in the creek.

We explored the grounds and Sara napped before driving the few miles to her brother's home for dinner.

The next day, we hiked briefly before a bout of dizziness hit Sara. We sat for a bit, but I could tell she was feeling less than comfortable with the fast-changing terrain and the elevation of more than 7,000 feet. The last thing either of us wanted, or needed, was a fall.

The day was everything the Colorado Department of Tourism touts about the state. The cloudless sky was so sharply blue you would swear it was painted on a backdrop. The abundant sunshine was quickly warming the spring air, and we drove southeast through the Arkansas River canyon. The runoff from the snow on the high mountains was beginning, and the river was roaring along, sparkling in the sun.

It was a good day for Sara, too. After the brief dizzy spell, she had bounced back and was more lucid and engaged than she had been in recent memory. We shared stories, recounted memories, laughed, and talked as we used to. It felt like the times we drove through the mountains during our college days.

We had been laughing and kidding one another when I came to a sweeping corner in the canyon I knew well. As I peered ahead and down the road, I noticed a sign that said, "Falling Rock." I glanced in the mirrors and started to slow the rental car. One of Sara's few fears in life was driving in the mountains and having to worry about a rock bouncing down a mountainside toward the car. We knew it could be serious; people had lost their lives in such incidents.

But it was something I always kidded her about and I was chiding her again as I pulled the car to the side of the road. There was just enough space for me to park, and I looked behind me as one of the tens of thousands of pickup trucks in Colorado roared past. I walked around the car, opened her door, and helped her out.

"I have to get a picture of you next to that sign," I said, smiling as I steadied her stance.

"All right," she said with a smile, giving in to my somewhat warped sense of humor. "I get it."

She stood with the sign in the background and I snapped the shutter a couple times to get the shot. I quickly moved back to her side and steadied her as we walked back to the car.

"Are you satisfied?" she said, feigning agitation with my request before she smiled again.

"I had to have that picture," I said. "You're always so rationale, so put together. This is such a departure from that for you, and I wanted it as a reminder that we all have our anxieties."

She laughed at my explanation.

"Don't give me your PR spiel. You're just giving me a hard time," she said with a laugh. "Just admit it. You've been doing it for thirty-five years and I'd never expect it to be any other way."

I looked at her as a tractor-trailer roared past and shook the car. My sense of love for her swept over me.

"Thanks for doing this. I love you so much," I said to her and leaned in to give her a kiss.

Tears formed in her eyes and mine. We kissed and held one another for several moments. Traffic buzzed by, oblivious to the special moment occurring in our car. Another big truck zipped closely by and brought us back to the reality of our situation. I pulled back and looked at Sara.

"We better get going before one of these guys sideswipes us," I said and we pulled back onto the highway.

Sara and I continued our thoughtful chatter as our journey continued. It was a comfort, a throwback to the "normal" life that seemed a very distant memory. I savored that day as life played out and the months passed. I continue to do so to this day. It was the last time our banter was on that high a level, and it was something I'd missed very deeply.

We continued east along the river, dropping slowly from the higher altitude, and eventually we were back at 5,000 feet as we drove into Pueblo. The contrasts of Colorado were playing out before us. We arrived at Sara's sister's ranch in the middle of the afternoon. The temperature was in the mideighties and the barren landscape was dusty and flat. There were vistas on the 30,000-acre ranch showing nothing on the horizon—not a tree, a power pole, or a house. Nothing but the earth rising to meet the sky. It was such a dramatic change from the spectacle of the Rockies where we had spent our previous day.

We were there a couple of nights and enjoyed our visit. Then we caught up with another friend for dinner on Denver's south side and, the next morning, drove to the airport for our return to Detroit.

As we made our way to the gate, I could tell the whirlwind week had taken a very real toll on Sara. She was less steady on her feet and I saw fatigue in her face. She let out a big sigh as we settled into the seats at the Northwest gate area.

"I've had a wonderful time," she said, the weariness in her voice coming through, "but I am really ready to get home. I miss our house, our bed, the dogs. And I can't wait to see Jen. Even as hard as it is to see her in Children's Home, I can't wait to see her again. And while everything has gone all right, I worry about being away from my doctors."

She stopped for several seconds and looked down at her hands, sitting folded in her lap, before she continued. She spoke of how fortunate we were to have the medical team we had, how they had become part of our family. I agreed, although I would have preferred to have never met them.

We boarded the plane and soon were airborne, winging our way back toward the Great Lakes. Sara's head, cancerous tumors and all, fell onto my left shoulder as she slipped into sleep. I looked out the small window and wondered what the next few months would hold. It was a question that never left my mind and, at times like this, it filled my head, and heart. I had spent so many hours and days in airplanes, winging my way around the world. They took me away from the day-to-day issues I faced with Sara and Jenny. But, as difficult as it could be to deal with those struggles, I always would have preferred to be there for them, and Andrew.

I had evolved to be a man with a vast array of emotions. I constantly worried about our finances. It was at the forefront of a sense of anxiety that regularly rose and fell. Generally, I was able to keep the anxiety at a low level and in check. But there were moments when it bubbled up and I would wonder how I would handle everything as it played out. The sense of uncertainty I knew was coming created apprehension, too, but I usually was able to push it to the back of my mind. On some level, I wondered just how the ever-growing anxiety was impacting my overall health.

A few wispy clouds were off in the distance as I thought about the trip that was ending. We had so many terrific friends and memories in Colorado. I truly wondered, though, if these were the last Colorado memories Sara and I would ever create. Tears rolled from my eyes as I watched the world pass by at more than five hundred miles per hour, and I had to fight back the desire to start a real cry.

We returned to Troy and it was nice to spend the next few weeks around the house. Not having to go to work provided a terrific break from my crazy schedule and it had given me the time to do a few things around the house, including finishing our basement. I did some wallpapering, too, to make the space more inviting. It served as a good place to display the many pieces of sports and entertainment art and memorabilia I had collected during my days doing sports, entertainment and events. We also wanted space in which we could display family photos, and I worked with Sara to get our many pictures framed. We placed them on one large wall and it was a nice montage of our parents, brothers, sisters, nieces, and nephews.

Among other things, that finished space gave Sara a place where she could work on her scrapbooking projects. While her goal was the completion of a scrapbook that featured our family, and several for each of the kids, I knew Sara well enough to understand she saw this as a way to stay busy and maintain her motor skills. Creating the scrapbooks was mentally and physically challenging and stimulating, and Sara knew very well she needed to try to maintain her dexterity and mental acuity. She alluded to that but never directly said it when we talked about finishing the space.

Having completed the basement, and with the weather getting warmer, I moved my focus outside. On the back of the house, we had a very large deck and it was in need of some attention. Sara wanted to stain it a redwood color. I'd never been a fan of staining and pushed back at first. But it became obvious she felt strongly about it, while I was somewhat ambivalent.

It was not unlike our latest automobile purchase. In 2000, we decided to replace Sara's aging car. Even in the midst of her chemo treatments, she found the energy to car shop, and found the one she wanted—a silver 1999 Chrysler LHS. I was not overly enthused about it. It seemed to be a nice car, had low miles, and was in good shape. But I didn't really care that much for it because it seemed a bit too boat-like for me.

But she wanted it. And I knew that this could very well be the last time she identified and expressed a desire for a specific car. I decided I would not stand in the way of her getting it. I checked it out a bit more thoroughly and agreed to the purchase.

Sara had enjoyed driving it in the ensuing years, but, in 2002, I was becoming concerned about her driving ability. I noticed she was beginning to lose some of her dexterity behind the wheel. It came to a head when she was driving down a nearby neighborhood street and, with her passenger-side mirror, clipped the driver-side mirror of a parked car. It amazed me she could get that close without actually hitting

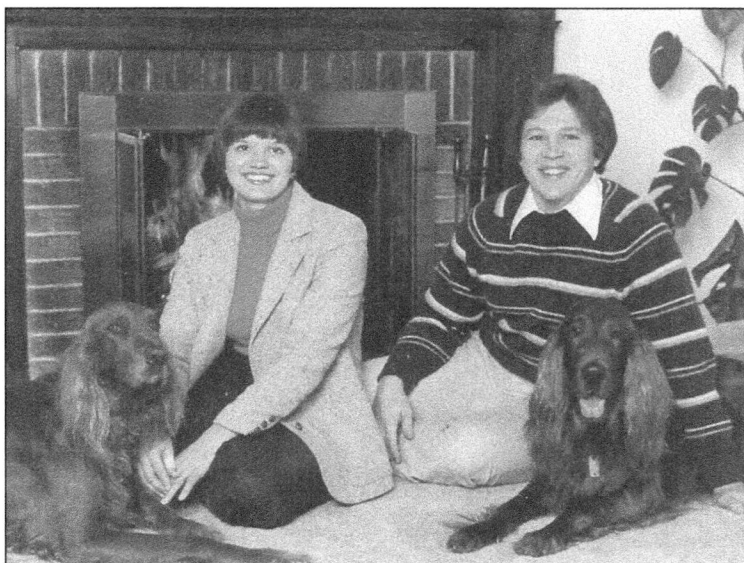
Sara and Ron with Irish Setters, 1980

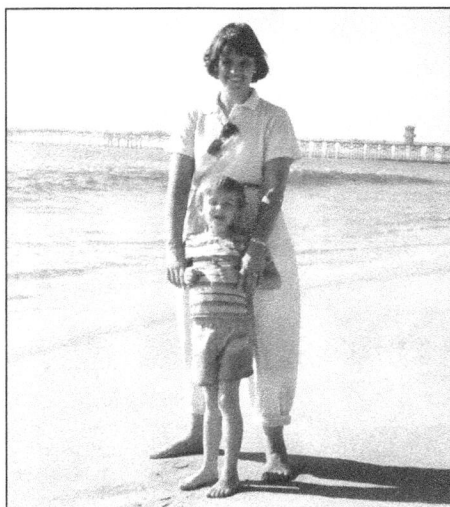
Sara and Andrew, Huntington Beach,
California, 1986

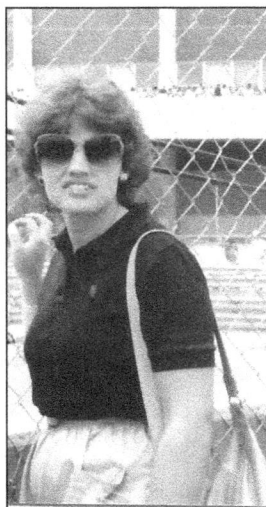
Sara, 1998

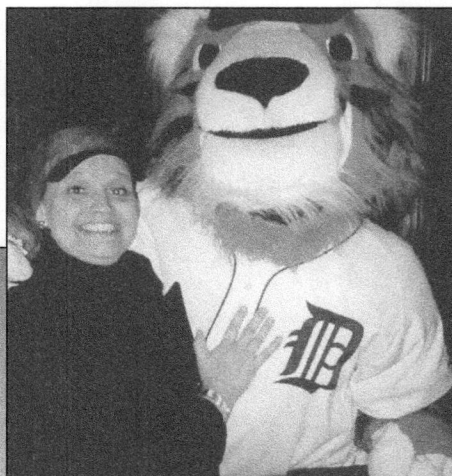
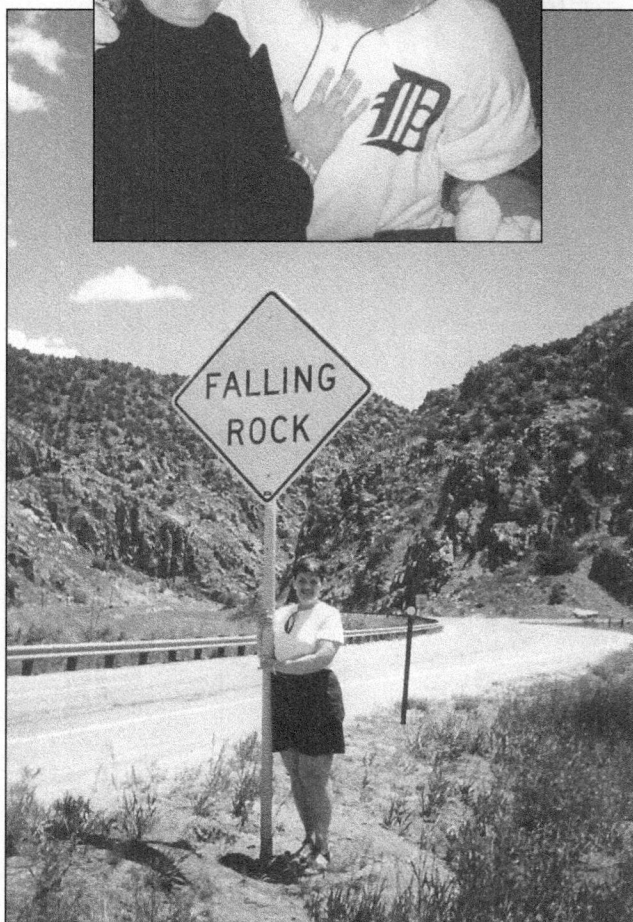

Top: Sara at a Detroit Tigers game, 2002
Bottom: Sara in Arkansas River Canyon west of Pueblo, 2003

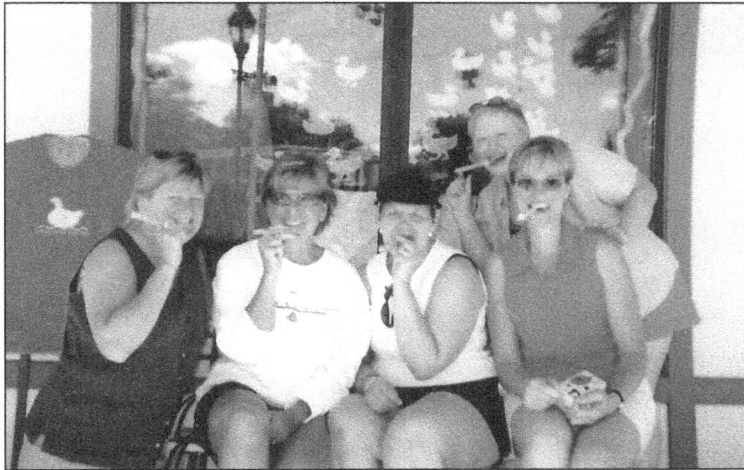

Sara and high school friends in northern Michigan, 2002

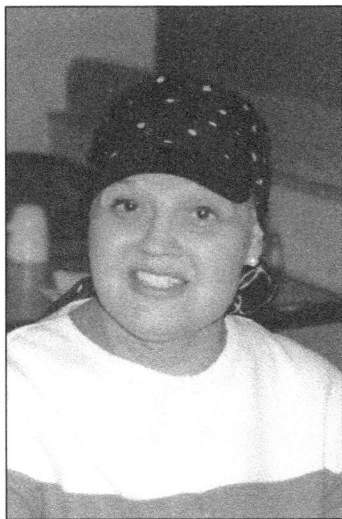

Sara, 2000

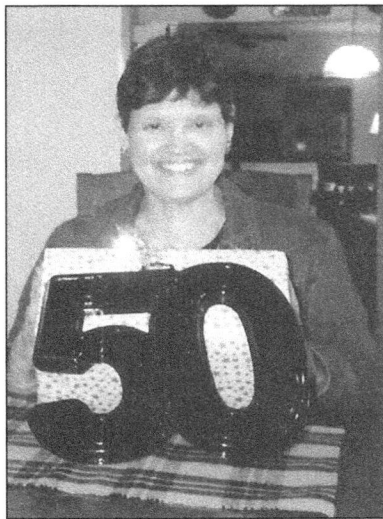

Sara on her 50th birthday, 2002

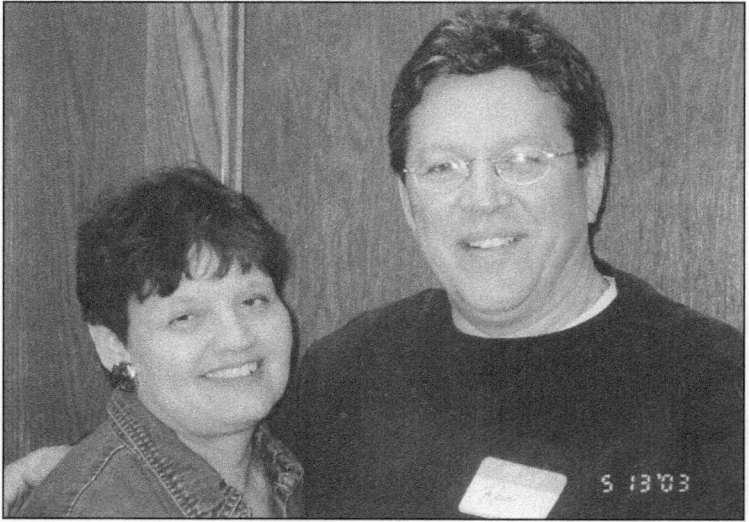

Sara and Ron, 2003

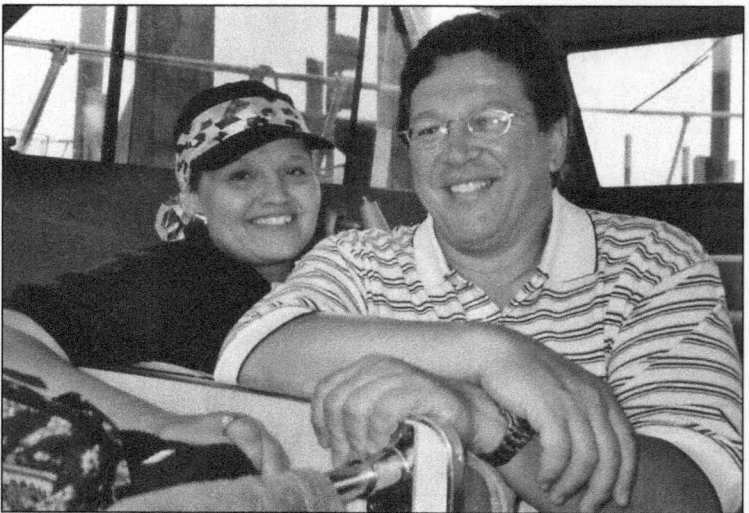

Sara and Ron at Put-in-Bay, Ohio, 2003

the car. There was no other damage, but it prompted me to suggest that she limit, and eventually eliminate, her driving. She reluctantly agreed to scale back, but not without disappointment and displeasure.

I felt bad about my suggestion that she stop driving. I knew it was one of the core elements of her feeling independent. But I couldn't allow her to hurt either herself or someone else.

I kept that in mind as I considered her request about the deck. I really didn't want to stain it. I knew it would require staining every year after and I thought that an unnecessary task. But it was something that would please her, and since she really wanted it, I relented and the deck soon had a red tint to it.

At the same time, we had been talking about how nice it would be to have a place on a lake. As kids, we had spent many days at small, inland lakes in southeast Michigan. Since moving to Troy, we loved our annual week at Round Lake, about two hours from our home. Sara insisted we share a day with each of our families, inviting them to join us, play in the water, have a barbeque, and play yard games like volleyball, badminton, and bocce ball. Living at the lake was something we had discussed prior to Sara's metastases, but as the reality of her battle with cancer was playing out, I knew it would not become a reality.

But that didn't mean we couldn't be there on a daily basis at our Troy home. As part of the deck renovation and staining project, I had thought hard about how I could bring the lake to our backyard. I mapped out a plan that would result in a dock, similar to those found in front of cottages on a lake, becoming part of our yard.

The previous owners had built one of those large, wooden play structures in the corner of the yard. I had disassembled most of it and placed a porch swing where the original swings had hung. Sara loved the swing and spent much time there, especially as she went through her chemo.

My idea was to build a walkway—the "dock"—from the deck out to the swing. Sara loved the concept and encouraged me to build it. After completing it, I stained it to match the deck. Sara was giddy as I finished it, and I felt great about having created a meaningful symbol that pleased her.

Our summer passed and we spent a good amount of time determining who we would see, our routes, and where we would stay along the way on our second planned trip. We left in early September and drove north on I-75 through the changing beauty of Michigan's woods and forests.

We reached the northern tip of the Lower Peninsula in the early afternoon and crossed the spectacular Mackinac suspension bridge. We came off the bridge into St. Ignace and took a ferry to Mackinac Island, a small resort island on which cars are not allowed. It is truly a step back in time and its Grand Hotel was featured in the movie *Somewhere in Time*, which starred Christopher Reeve and Christopher Plummer. We took a tour by horse-drawn carriage and strolled through the small town that sits above the marina and is well-known for its candies and fudge.

After spending the night, we reboarded the high-speed ferry back to the mainland. The wind had come up overnight and the ride was rougher than we had experienced the previous afternoon. Sara held me tightly as the massive catamaran sped and bounced across the water toward St. Ignace. She admitted to being nauseous and was afraid she might vomit before we made it back to shore. I did all I could to distract her and, somehow, she managed to make it. But her face was ghastly white and she couldn't wait to get on solid ground.

"That tumor is doing its work on my vestibular system," she said. "I was so queasy and really thought I would get sick."

I tried to change the focus as we got into our car. "We have a beautiful drive ahead of us. Let's focus on that."

Sara agreed, but I could feel her angst and knew she wished she were at home, in her bed. The boat ride had sapped her energy, in addition to making her feel sick.

Once we were back in the car, she fell asleep almost immediately and slept hard for a couple of hours. I drove alongside the northwest edge of Lake Michigan, enjoying the drive and the vistas above the shimmering water. Late in the afternoon, we arrived in Green Bay, Wisconsin, where we spent the evening visiting with a therapist friend of Sara's and her family.

The next day, we had a much easier and shorter drive, motoring south through Wisconsin until we came to Mequon, where we had lived before moving to Michigan. We arrived at the home of the Hennicks, our longtime friends and neighbors.

It was great to catch up with Mike and Elena. As it had in Colorado, our conversation turned to how we were coping. They told us they thought of us often and wished they could do more to help. It felt great to have their genuine affection and support, and it also gave us another opportunity to share the message that cancer and other life problems don't have to bring a couple or a family to a screeching halt. We didn't pretend that it was easy for us, but we really thought it was important for our friends to know that staying positive and closely connected as a couple made it life affirming instead of overwhelming.

I spoke to the importance of acceptance, too. While it was often difficult to get there, I reiterated the importance, and satisfaction, of doing so.

As our conversations continued, Mike and I talked about my career and how the year away might affect my ability to land my next position. I told him I'd been preoccupied with Sara and her care, but I'd also begun to sniff around the job market. My inclination was to stay in sports. I wasn't sure where or with whom, but I was growing a bit restless.

"I don't know what I'll do but I'm probably most interested in getting another job in sports," I told him. "Maybe I'll remain in motorsports. The auto guys are always looking for people to do marketing and PR for their racing efforts. And I have quite a few connections there. I've also talked to some agencies, so I could go in that direction. That's one thing I've never done in my career and it holds some interest for me."

It was great to have the conversation with him, and it reinforced my need to generate an income. That reality was gnawing at my being and kicked around in my mind. I'd worked to maintain my relationships and contacts in the large network I had developed over the years. I was convinced it would serve me well. But I loved being Sara's primary caregiver and I did not want to, nor would I, relinquish that responsibility. It had brought us closer together than we had ever been. Still, the need for an income meant I would soon have to begin working again.

After a couple days, we left Wisconsin behind and spent a night with one of our best friends from high school and her husband. Beth and Dan McCormick live a block off Michigan Avenue in downtown Chicago, a far cry from the solitude and rural beauty of the Upper Peninsula where we had been only a few days before.

Beth had always been one of Sara's best friends, and she held a special place in my heart, too. She had been my girlfriend when we were in eighth grade. We had made a real effort to stay in touch over the years, and it was always terrific to get together with the two of them.

We left Chicago the following morning, drove south out of downtown, around the southern end of Lake Michigan, through northwestern Indiana, and into southern Michigan. We had one more stop; we would spend the evening in Kalamazoo with Andrew. It was great to see him in his environment. He had become such a terrific young man. His AmeriCorps experience had matured him and prepared him well for college. He was very focused on his studies and seemed to be truly enjoying his college experience. Western Michigan was a good state university and Andrew was maintaining a strong grade point average.

He had also met a woman and the two seemed very taken with one another. They spent most of their time together and their relationship was becoming quite serious. She was from Clarkston, a far northern suburb of Detroit, about a half hour from our Troy home.

We had a great evening with them and headed back to our suburban Detroit home in the morning. Our drive around Lake Michigan had racked up more than 1,200 miles.

It had been a fun-filled week, but I could tell Sara was very ready to get home.

"I don't know how many more trips I can make," she said. "I know how much it means to you to get out, see people, and do these things. And I really appreciate your planning everything and making it happen. But it wears me down and my energy level seems to become less and less with every passing day."

"I know. I'm happy you've been willing to make the effort you have to do this," I said. "For me, and for the people who want to see you, it's been great to have you out here. But I do recognize how it affects you."

Sara interrupted me.

"I love seeing everyone—you know that," she said. "But, as you know, what I say about saving my energy is very true. It's important for me to not wear myself out. I've come closer to doing that, at times, than anyone—even you—realizes. I don't want to end up back in the hospital."

I got the message loud and clear.

"Understood," I said. "I'm glad you told me, though. I don't want to make this any harder on us—especially you—than it needs to be."

We each knew that nothing more needed to be said, except that we loved one another. And even that didn't need to be said. But we said it. The hum of the car heading east on I-94 became the prominent sound. A few minutes later, Sara was again sleeping.

CHAPTER

12

While I savored the moments Sara and I were spending together, I was also beginning to feel the void that came with not working. I was getting restless.

The change had been dramatic. I was used to working twelve-hour days, being gone for nearly a week at a time, traveling with the circus that was IndyCar racing. The creative juices I applied to work were pent up, and I was beginning to wonder what I would do next. When I wasn't helping Sara and taking her to her many appointments, I had tentatively begun searching for my next career stop.

The cancer in Sara's head was slowly changing. The tumor, which had not been fully radiated in the stereotactic procedure, was growing and occasionally would do so in a manner that affected her ability to function. We worried about it pushing on the tissue near her brain stem. The pressure could result in a variety of potential outcomes, all negative.

Jenny remained at Children's Home of Detroit, and while making some progress, was often difficult to be around. She didn't seem to be as volatile, thanks to a combination of therapy and the introduction of medicines that brought her blood chemical levels back to more normal levels. Her impulsivity seemed to have lessened, but she could still become difficult in a relatively short period of time. Still, the improvement allowed her to come home on weekends with more regularity, something Sara and I looked forward to.

One weekend in early November, Sara seemed more tired than usual. I left her at home on Friday afternoon to go to CHD to pick up Jenny.

"How's Mom doing?" Jenny asked as we began our way home. She seemed cheery and more engaged than we often found her.

"Mom's doing all right," I said. "She's been more tired than usual the past couple of days but otherwise, she's been good. I think we need to let her rest a bit more than we usually do this weekend so she can rebuild her energy."

Jenny seemed to be thinking about what I'd just said for several moments before she responded.

"Dad? How long before Mom is going to die?"

It was an unexpected question. Jenny was generally concerned about Sara but didn't ask such pointed questions.

"Why do you ask, Jen?" I said, trying to gather my thoughts.

"I've just been thinking about it," she said. "I don't know why."

I glanced toward her as we turned off Mound Road and headed west on 18 Mile Road.

"I wish we could know more about how this will play out," I said, trying to avoid getting her even more concerned. "It's kind of like your illness and time at CHD. We don't really know."

"But I'm not going to die. Mom will, won't she?"

I hesitated but answered. "We don't know, Jen. Cancer is a funny thing. Sometimes it wins; other times it doesn't. Mom's cancer is very serious. We just need to stay focused on what we know today and enjoy the time we have with her. Will she eventually die? We all do. Do we ever know when? No, we don't."

Jenny was quiet and I could see she was tearing up a bit.

"I don't want Mom to die," she said. "I hope she is here forever."

"Me too," I said. "We just have to be patient and wait to see what happens."

Trying to change the subject, I mentioned that I had spoken to Andrew the night before. Jenny took the bait and asked about her brother.

When we arrived at home, I turned to Jenny, gave her a hug, and said, "Jen? Let's have a good weekend, okay?"

"Okay, Dad," she said. "I'll be good."

We went inside and found Sara in the kitchen, looking out the window over the sink. I asked her if she was okay as she turned to greet us.

"Yeah, I'm fine," she replied in a flat, almost monotone voice that was unlike her.

Jenny moved toward her and the two hugged. Sara seemed a little distant, but I dismissed it as a side effect of the steroid she was taking. She'd had another brain scan at the end of the previous week and it indicated the tumor had grown. Her doctors put her on a steroid in pill form. I never knew how she would respond to the medicine, but it often made her sleep less, which, in turn, could make her edgy and terse.

We went out to dinner, watched a movie back at home, and then went upstairs for bed about 10:45. Shortly thereafter, Sara went to Jenny's room to say good night. Sara had been unusually quiet for most of the night, but I could hear the sound of them talking as I crawled into bed.

A few minutes passed and Jenny suddenly appeared at my bedside.

"Dad," she said, pushing on my shoulder, "I'm afraid of Mom. She's saying some strange things."

I quickly focused on Jenny and asked her to repeat herself.

"Mom is acting weird," she said. "I'm scared. I want to go back to CHD."

Now I was wide awake and sat up in bed. I looked to the open bedroom door where Sara stood, then got up and went to my closet to put on a shirt. Jenny stayed behind me as I approached Sara.

"Are you all right?" I asked her.

At first, she didn't respond. After a few seconds she said she was fine. But when I asked her about what Jenny had said, she had a strange and vacant look on her face and didn't respond. I wasn't sure what to do. Jenny remained behind me and pulled at my sleeve.

"Dad. I want to go back to CHD. Can we go? *Now*?"

Sara, in turn, responded by saying that Jenny was making things up. I was stuck in the middle and confused. I wondered what Sara had said, but she wouldn't say and Jenny refused to tell me. The one thing I did know was that Jenny was frightened.

"Okay, Jen," I said. "We'll take you back."

I gathered up Jenny's stuff. Sara had not yet slipped out of her jeans and sweater and I managed to get her downstairs. I called ahead to Children's Home to let them know we were returning. Jenny crawled into the backseat of the car and Sara sat silently beside me as we drove to the facility.

When we arrived at CHD a few minutes later, I turned to Sara and asked her if she was doing all right. She turned toward me, said nothing, and just stared. Jenny and I walked up the sidewalk to the psych hospital and were greeted by a staff member. I specifically conveyed to her that this had nothing to do with Jenny's behavior, and she said she would make note of it in Jenny's chart.

Jenny seemed genuinely disturbed by the experience she had with her mom.

"Dad, Mom was saying things that scared me," she said. "She is just acting really strange. Thank you for bringing me back."

I hugged her and told her it would be okay. She looked around me and out to the car before she walked into the hospital with the staff member.

I returned to the car and sat down behind the steering wheel. I turned to say something to Sara but she screamed at me before I could speak.

"I can't believe you aren't supporting me! You're taking Jenny's word over mine? I can't believe you would do that. I want you to take me to Marilyn's *right now.*"

I was stunned. I tried to calm her as we started on our way home. Obviously, something was going on in Sara's head that was taking her way outside her normal frame of reference.

"I don't know what you mean," I said, trying to remain calm. "I don't understand what you're talking about."

Sara continued her ranting and yelling at me. In the thirty-five years I had known her, she had never acted in this way.

She again told me to take her to see Marilyn, her best friend. I stayed silent and kept driving. Suddenly, she reached for the steering wheel. I stopped her hand before she could grab it. I made a U-turn and headed south.

Sara immediately started yelling again.

"What are you doing? Turn around! I want to go to Marilyn's and you need to take me there now."

I was doing all I could to stay calm and I remained focused on the road to avoid eye contact.

"Sara, you aren't yourself and I'm taking you to Beaumont where they can check you out."

"I'm fine and don't need to go to the hospital," she snapped. "Take me to Marilyn's. Now!"

I drove to the hospital as quickly as I could. Sara's ranting didn't subside for a couple of miles. I stopped acknowledging her and she turned quiet. A red light brought us to a stop. Ahead loomed a welcome sight: Beaumont. The light changed and we were soon sitting in the familiar semicircular driveway in front of the emergency room entrance.

Sara sat still in the car and I wondered if she would resist getting into the wheelchair being pushed toward the car by a security person. I told him Sara needed to see a doctor but that she might resist getting out of the car. He nodded and opened the door. Sara hesitated but slowly emerged and sat in the chair. She glared at me as she was turned toward the entrance door and pushed into the ER.

We went through the admission process we knew all too well. Sara refused to answer many of the questions asked by the admissions person. An orderly wheeled her back to a draped examination area, and we sat for a few minutes before a nurse came by and got her vital signs and quizzed us on why we were there. Sara sat silently as I recounted the bizarre behavior I had seen the past few hours. The nurse took it all down and soon a doctor drew open the drape.

"So tell me why you're here," he said as he perused the chart.

I started to speak and he stopped me.

"I'd like to hear what Sara has to say first," he said.

Sara looked up at him, then at me.

"Thank you," she said, glaring at me again. "I don't know why we're here. I told him I wanted to go to be with my friend Marilyn and he wouldn't take me."

The doctor looked at the chart, made a couple of notes, and then asked me to accompany him out of the exam area. We walked to a quiet place on the other side of the ER. It was no surprise that the place was bustling. It was Saturday night in a major metropolitan hospital.

"Have you seen this kind of behavior from Sara before?" the doctor asked.

"No," I said. "My daughter was afraid of Sara, something I've never seen before. It was something Sara said to her."

"Did she tell you what Sara said?" he asked.

"No. She didn't want to talk about it," I replied.

"And this yelling at you. It's not typical of her?"

"Absolutely not. Sara is always calm and reasonable," I said. "But she wasn't on the way over here. She rarely gets agitated, but she has been the past couple of hours. She recently started taking steroids again because of the tumor in her brain and I wonder if that has anything to do with it. When she's on steroids, she often doesn't sleep much and her personality becomes more abrupt and confrontational. Do you think the steroids could be the cause of this?"

The doctor continued reviewing the chart as he gathered his thoughts.

"I don't know that the steroids have anything to do with this," he said. "It's certainly possible, but my experience is that steroids don't cause this kind of thing. With the ongoing change in her tumor, it may be putting pressure on her brain tissue and causing this. I'd like you to stay here for the next few hours so we can review Sara's history, take a look at her latest scans, and observe her behavior. We'll let Dr. Decker's office know, but I would be surprised if they want to do anything more than we're planning to do."

I thanked him and returned to the curtained exam room where Sara was sitting on the gurney that served as an exam table.

"I want to leave. I'm tired and want to be in my own bed. Why did you bring me here? I feel fine," Sara said, still angry with me.

"Sara, you've been acting strangely," I said. "Whatever you said to Jenny disturbed her greatly, and you were screaming at me about not supporting you and wanting to go to Marilyn's house."

I could see confusion in her eyes. I stepped closer and hugged her.

"It's my job to take care of you," I said as I held her. "When you behave as you have, I wouldn't be doing my job if I didn't bring you here."

Sara looked up and into my face, and I could clearly tell she was confused and struggling with what was happening.

"I'm tired," she said, and she leaned back against the gurney.

I knew it was time to step back to give her space. I sat down next to the gurney and Sara dozed off. I, too, nodded off and slept off and on over the next several hours in the ER.

A nurse came in about 5:00 a.m. and checked Sara's vitals again. Another doctor examined Sara about 8:00 a.m. and didn't have anything new to add to her status. Sara was getting restless and so was I. Her level of agitation had diminished overnight and we were both ready to go home.

A nurse told us at about 9:30 that Sara would soon be discharged, and we left about an hour later.

The drive home was quiet for a time. Then Sara again asked why I had taken her to the hospital. I repeated what I had said the previous night.

She listened closely but chose not to respond, and we soon pulled into the garage and went into the house.

The dogs greeted us and I let them out into the backyard to relieve themselves.

"I'm going up to take a shower," Sara said as I opened the door to go outside. "I have to meet Marilyn for lunch at 1:00."

I stood in the warming morning air and waited a few minutes for the dogs to do their business before reentering the kitchen.

I discovered Sara standing at the sink, looking out the window into the backyard as she was when Jenny and I arrived the prior evening.

"Are you okay?" I asked her.

She didn't respond but continued to stare out the window.

I asked her again. And then again. She failed to acknowledge me.

I approached her and she turned toward me. Her look startled me. It was faraway, vacant. She pivoted from the sink and started to walk away. I tried to stop her but she gently pushed her way past me and headed out of the kitchen and up the stairs.

I followed her closely as she ascended the narrow stairway. I spoke again to engage her as we headed upstairs, but the disconnected look remained and she did not respond. She came to the top of the stairs and turned into our bedroom and remained unresponsive. I thought of the oppositional attitude she'd had over the past several hours, but this was different. She was no longer angry about having been taken to the hospital. She was, literally, checked out but on her feet, moving as if all was okay.

But it wasn't.

I followed her into the bathroom and, suddenly, she spoke.

"I'm going to get in the shower," she said, turning toward me and looking puzzled. "Why are you following me?"

I was stunned. Just moments before, she had been in a zombie-like trance.

"How do you feel?" I said. "Are you okay?"

"I'm fine," she replied, an edge to her voice. "Why do you keep asking me that?"

"You just walked up here from the kitchen without saying a word to me after I asked you a question several times," I replied.

"I don't know what you are talking about," she said. "I just need to get cleaned up so I can meet Marilyn."

This was getting more and more strange by the moment.

"All I know is that you were walking up the stairs and into the bedroom, in an almost zombie-like state, and I kept asking you questions and you didn't answer me. Are you sure you're all right?"

I could tell by her body language that she was getting impatient with my questions. But I needed to know why this was happening.

"I don't know what you're talking about," she said again as she began to undress to get in the shower.

She pulled her top off and her demeanor changed again. Her eyes were open but she came to a standstill. I once again asked her if she was all right. No response.

I led her to the bed and sat her down on its edge. She sat, not saying a thing. I tried several times over the next couple of minutes to get her to respond with no luck. Suddenly, she stood, walked back to the bathroom, and continued to undress.

"Sara, you just zoned out again, like you did before. Are you sure you're okay?"

She looked at me with disbelief.

"I just told you I'm fine," she almost snapped at me. "Why do you keep asking me if I'm okay? I'm all right."

I was beginning to get panicky. I focused, locking in on my logical mind, and recounted the situation to make sure I wasn't missing something. She was completely disengaged, for a few minutes at a time. I thought about how she was totally oblivious to me or my questions. It lasted a few minutes before she snapped back to reality, responding as if nothing had happened. Her voice broke my train of thought.

"I'm getting in the shower," she said from the bathroom.

I was afraid to leave her alone. I wasn't sure what was happening, but it seemed these were some sort of seizure-like episodes. As much as I did not want to suggest it, I was thinking we had to go back to the hospital. I knew she would become completely obstinate if I mentioned that, but I was fast becoming convinced she needed to be seen as soon as possible. I also figured that getting Marilyn involved would help since Sara was looking forward to seeing her. I pulled out my cell phone, rang her up, and described the situation. She said she would be right over.

About twenty minutes later, she was at the door and I left Sara, who had slipped into another trance, to let Marilyn in.

"Marilyn, this is one of the weirdest things I've ever seen," I said as we bounded up the stairs. "One minute, she's perfectly normal, talking about getting ready to meet you for lunch, and the next minute she's completely zoned out. She won't respond at all."

Sara was seated on the edge of the bed, wet from her shower. I announced that Marilyn was here to see her. Marilyn spoke to her, but Sara was in the midst of another episode and didn't respond.

We helped Sara to her feet and dried her off. I pulled her robe around her and Marilyn tried speaking to her, but the effort elicited no response. Marilyn looked at me and agreed that we should get Sara to the hospital as soon as possible.

Sara remained silent for the next minute before she abruptly spoke.

"Marilyn, what are you doing here?" Sara asked, a look of confusion on her face.

"I just came by a little early to help you get ready," Marilyn said. "Are you feeling okay? You seem to be going in and out a bit."

Sara looked at her, confusion coming across her face.

"I told Ron that I'm fine," she said. "I don't know why you keep asking me about this."

Marilyn said that she thought we should go back to the hospital so the doctors could check out what was going on with Sara.

"Marilyn," Sara said. "I was just at the hospital. They kept me overnight and everything is okay."

I stayed silent, knowing that my intervention would most likely cause Sara to escalate.

"You keep blanking out," Marilyn said. "I'm not sure what we should do. But I'm worried about you and I think a doctor needs to see you."

Almost on cue, Sara again went into her trance-like state. She didn't try to walk off or do anything but sit still on the edge of the bed.

"Marilyn, these episodes are coming more frequently, and they seem to be lasting slightly longer each time," I said. "The first one lasted only a minute or so, but the last one was the fourth or fifth one and it went on for more than two minutes. I'll time this one to see, but I'm getting really worried."

Marilyn was trying to stay calm, too. It was good that we could double-team Sara, and we helped each other remain composed as we tried to get Sara's agreement on going back to Beaumont.

"Let's get her dressed and to the car. I'll sit in the backseat with her and keep her occupied," Marilyn said. "I think this is serious. I agree that we need to get her to Beaumont as quickly as we can."

I nodded and continued to pull Sara's top over her head. Marilyn worked to get Sara's jeans on and then slipped on her shoes. By the time we finished, Sara was back with us, asking what we were doing. I let Marilyn do the talking because it seemed to agitate Sara less.

"Let's get you to the hospital to see a doctor," Marilyn said. "These blackouts you're having really concern me. Let's just get you back there so they can check on you, okay?"

Sara seemed confused but reluctantly agreed.

I went downstairs to get the car ready, and Marilyn led Sara down the steps. We wanted to get her into the car before she zoned out again. Once the three of us were in the car, I headed back to Beaumont. During the drive, Sara experienced two more seizure-like episodes and was just coming out of the second as we pulled into the ER drive.

A security person met us and, along with Marilyn, helped Sara into a wheelchair. I parked and hurried back to the ER admitting area. Sara and Marilyn were nowhere to be seen and I walked directly into the ER. I recognized the nurse who had come on in the early morning during our previous visit. She was taking Sara's vital signs as I walked to the side of the movable bed.

"I couldn't believe it when I saw your wife back here," the nurse told me. "I'm really sorry you had to come back."

Marilyn had started telling her about the episodes and I filled in the blanks. Sara sat, looking vacantly into the distance. She was clearly becoming worn down by the constant seizure-like periods. What was worrisome was that they were growing in length. Over the next hour, Sara spent more than twenty minutes having episodes.

While the staff had been relatively unconcerned the night before, they were concerned now. A doctor came by in short order and ordered an EEG to monitor Sara's brainwave activity. A technician arrived in just a few minutes and connected the leads to Sara's skull. It didn't take long before the verdict was in. As we had suspected, Sara was having some sort of seizure activity.

The doctor viewed the output from the test and admitted Sara to the hospital. As usual, she was going to be placed on the seventh floor. They soon wheeled her away and continued to monitor her brainwaves as she groggily came to, then, in a couple minutes, went into another seizure.

Marilyn and I followed the orderly who wheeled her into the semi-private room. There was no one in the room's other bed, and Marilyn and I settled in while the orderly, a nurse, and another technician tended to Sara.

The amount of time Sara was spending in a seizure state had expanded to nearly half of each hour and was showing no signs of abating. A doctor soon came by and I asked him what was next.

"We're not certain, but it appears Sara's tumor is causing problems by pushing on tissue in her brain," he said. "We'll get in touch with Dr. Decker's office and let them know Sara's status. We'll continue to monitor her and see what happens"

Sara would remain in the hospital the next several days. I called Andrew after things settled down, and he came to Troy to be with us. The uncertainty of the situation weighed heavily on all of us, and it was great we could be together. Sara's seizures were difficult to watch, and for a time, they dominated her being. On Sunday, she was in a seizure state for more minutes of each hour than not, and on Monday it increased, for a brief time, to more than forty-five minutes per hour.

She was being given drugs in an attempt to mitigate the situation and, fortunately, they did their job. By Tuesday, she began to return to her normal state. She was extremely tired after all the seizure activity. The doctors decided she should stay for another day. After determining that there didn't appear to be any permanent damage to her brain, Sara was discharged the following day.

As we drove home, I thought of the dozens of trips we had made to and from the hospital. This one was different. While we always had worries about Sara's health, we had just experienced a new and more significant event. Sara's behavior had dramatically changed for a few days. I wanted to talk about it with her, but I was certain such a discussion would be futile.

During the brief conversations we had about this episode, it was apparent she had no knowledge of what had gone on—or how she had behaved. I was frustrated by that because we had always been able to honestly and openly talk about things. I felt alone and wanted to talk through it with her. But I couldn't. That loneliness was, at times, nearly overwhelming.

I found myself thinking of Sara as she sat on the edge of the bed, dripping wet and zoned out. Even though it was difficult, I forced myself to ignore those images, deciding I couldn't go there. Those thoughts brought negativity to our life and, like Sara, I was learning I needed my energy to stay positive so I could be there for her.

We had reached, yet again, another level in our cancer journey. We had regularly redefined "normal" along the way. I preferred to look at it as the "new normal." Just when it felt as if we could settle into a routine, such as when Sara was doing her chemo treatments, our entire frame of reference would shift. It caused us to reset our thinking and approach, and it never really allowed us to feel like life was what we once perceived as "normal." The bottom line was that normal was a moving target and, over the final three years of Sara's life, it often moved with little or no notice or fanfare. Normal became a very subjective and often surreal place, one that had only one certainty: it would soon again change and we'd better be prepared to adapt because there was not much we could do to manage it.

The final few weeks of 2002 flew past. Jenny remained at Children's Home of Detroit while Andrew's quarter at Western Michigan was winding down.

Sara and I began to look ahead to the Thanksgiving and Christmas holidays. We planned Thanksgiving with my family in Troy. When Sara had the focus and energy, we also began gathering Christmas gifts for the kids. The Christmas season came and we spent time with Sara's family, as well as mine. It was great to have the kids around—Andrew home from college and Jenny home on a limited basis.

We found that Jenny could handle a few days at a time before she escalated and had a confrontation. When those instances arose, we would take her back to CHD. Had we not been able to take her back, I'm not sure how we would have managed. Balancing Sara's care with trying to keep Jenny in check was more than I was capable of handling.

Additionally, I was really feeling the pressure of not having a job. I had jumped back into the search, looking in earnest. The local economy was doing reasonably well, and I expected to land a local job in the PR and communications field. I connected with a couple of executive search firms and one, based in Atlanta, identified a handful of opportunities I found interesting. The one I most liked was based in Indianapolis, where I ended up interviewing for the position of director of public relations at the National Collegiate Athletic Association (NCAA).

I did a phone interview to start the process and made the cut. The result was a trip to Indianapolis to meet with the vice president of communications. She and I hit it off and I sensed the potential was good for landing the job.

She called me a few days later to say they wanted me to return and let me know who I would meet with. The list included Myles Brand, the President of the NCAA, as well as several of the senior leadership staff members. These were names I had seen for years. They were responsible, in part, for shaping the direction of college athletics. I learned it was down to me and one other candidate and was also told she would be comfortable with either of us in the job.

I was excited about the opportunity. Sara and I discussed it. I could sense she had some reservations, but we both knew I needed to land my next career stop sooner rather than later. This was a very high-profile position and one that approached, from an income standpoint, what I had been making at CART. Importantly for me, it would be something that I would truly love doing.

I returned to Indianapolis a few days later and the interview went very well. I was stoked about the potential as Sara and I talked over dinner once I was back in Troy.

"It was great," I said. "I met for almost an hour with (president) Myles Brand, and then with several members of his executive team. It went really well. This would be such a great opportunity. I would be in a position to help impact change in college sports. It's something I would love to do."

Sara listened intently. She smiled at my enthusiasm. I could tell she enjoyed seeing her fifty-one-year-old husband exude kid-like giddiness for a job. We got our food and I continued talking about the possibilities. As I was completing my meal, I noticed that Sara had just been moving her food around her plate. There was something on her mind.

"I've been doing all the talking," I said. "I can see, though, that something is on your mind."

Sara was hesitant but finally spoke.

"It's great to see how excited you are about this," she said. "I love your enthusiasm. You know that I have always been willing to go anywhere if it's best for our family. We've had so many wonderful adventures and I've loved every minute of it. I would never change any of that."

I could feel her apprehension and was waiting for the "but" I knew was coming.

"Our circumstances today are different," Sara added. "We both know where things are headed, and I want us to be able to enjoy our remaining time the best way we can. My doctors and Beaumont are here and I love them like family. And our families are close by, too."

She paused for what seemed to be a very long time.

"The bottom line is: I don't want to move again. I can't move again." Tears were forming in her eyes. "All of our support—friends and family—is here, and I just don't have the energy to move again. I know how much this means to you, and I really wish it was a different time in our lives so we could do it. It sounds like a wonderful job. But I just can't move."

I stood and moved to the other side of the booth to sit next to her. I put my arm around her and drew her close.

"I'm sorry," I said. "I feel so selfish in the way I've been talking about this. I didn't even think it would be an issue to move. We've always just pursued options like this and I guess I took it for granted. In the end, you're right. Our priority is to do what is best for our family. And right now, that is to care for you. If that means we stay here, then we stay here. You know we won't do it any other way. I'm just sorry I didn't see this."

Tears flowed down her cheeks and I could sense her relief after listening to my response.

"I hate it that you won't be able to go after this position. I know how much you want it. But I just can't move," she said again. She paused but then continued. "I'm sorry that I'm holding you back."

I immediately responded, pulling her closer to me. "You're not holding me back. There's always another job. I'll find something here. You know you're my priority now. I'll let the NCAA know I'm withdrawing from consideration."

She started to cry again.

"I could see how excited this possibility made you, and I didn't want to get in the way of that," she said, dabbing away her tears. "But as time went by and it became closer to becoming a reality, I knew that I couldn't leave. I just didn't want to say anything."

It was a pivotal moment in in our lives. I called the recruiter the next day and left a message for him. He didn't call back, which puzzled me. The following day, he got back to me and let me know the NCAA had made its decision. Obviously, it was not to offer me the job.

On the surface, my discussion with Sara became moot. However, underlying that conversation was the decision to stay in the Detroit area. Realistically, it ended up severely limiting the job opportunities I had. As I considered the options in Detroit, I knew it would be difficult to land something, but I also felt confident my background and experience would put me in a favorable position and I'd end up with something I truly wanted.

What I fully understood was that Sara needed me. And she needed the familiarity of Troy, her doctors, her friends, and our families. This time, my needs came second. She had, for all our married life, been the one who sacrificed. We had thoroughly discussed my career in sports early in our marriage and agreed on our plan. We both knew I would work long hours—nights and weekends—and would be away a lot. She was okay with that. We would move to advance my career. The result was that she had willingly given up positions as we moved. It was always done with the thought the change would lead to a greater family benefit. Better career opportunities. More income.

But now both of us recognized we had to optimize the time we had. We desperately needed one another during this difficult period. It was a mutual decision and I gladly accepted my role. I fully considered that as I surveyed the situation regarding potential career choices. The bottom line, though, was that something was going to have to come along. I would have to find a job. Soon. It was another stress and strain brought on by the cancer, and one not generally at the fore-front of the thoughts one has when dealing with a significant illness.

I dug into trying to find a local job. As I looked around the Motor City, I discovered few options. I looked at our dwindling savings and thought of my options. I filed for, and received, unemployment compensation. It was not something I'd expected to do, but I figured I'd paid into the system for more than thirty years; it was my time of need, and the safety net, meager as it was, was there for me.

As I completed the paperwork, I found it particularly ironic that in the time of greatest need, the system required you to pay taxes on an amount that didn't even come close to paying the bills. It truly felt like being kicked while I was down. Then, too, there was the stigma that comes with being on unemployment. Nonetheless, I was very grateful to get the check.

My job search continued into the late winter of 2003, and it was becoming noticeable that the economy in the metro-politan Detroit area was at the very front end of what would become the Great Recession. The US automotive companies were the eight hundred-pound gorilla in southeast Michigan, but were weakening with each passing month. Options in those fields were becoming fewer and fewer as days passed. And it trickled down to all kinds of businesses throughout the region.

However, the challenging work situation was just one of our concerns.

Jenny's stay at Children's Home of Detroit was coming to an end.

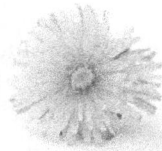

CHAPTER
13

Our Easter Seals representative came to our house in early January to discuss Jenny and the options for her ongoing treatment.

"You know," said Shari, the social worker who had Jenny's case and was a fabulous resource for us as we had navigated through the mental health system, "we've seen some encouraging signs with Jenny. She's made progress and we're thinking about what's next for her."

Sara and I listened intently to what she said but it didn't fully jibe with the reality we had seen with Jenny. The good thing was that she had gotten herself together to the point that she could come home on a regular basis for weekends and generally do okay. Over the next few weeks, we watched as Jenny did reasonably well during her passes. But we remained apprehensive about her being discharged.

By early February, the decision had been made. Jenny would be discharged later in the month and come home to live with us.

Sara and I were cautiously optimistic about how this would work. The window into the eventual outcome, though, came when, during one of her final sessions at CHD, Jenny said she had not progressed enough to be on the "outside." Sara and I spoke with the therapist and she indicated they felt they had given Jenny everything they could. She'd been there for eighteen months, received a lot of therapy, gotten on good meds, and made solid progress. But Jenny had said she wasn't ready, and I asked why she would say it if it was not true. The therapist explained that they often saw this with kids preparing to be discharged and stressed that they wouldn't be willing to release Jenny if they didn't think she was ready.

Sara and I had real concerns. We understood that Jenny could be trying to set expectations lower as she exited. But she seemed very genuine in her feelings about leaving CHD. Plus, we later learned, there had been pressure exerted on Easter Seals to move her out so another patient could move in. It's an ongoing problem in a country where mental health services, over the past several decades, have been decimated and patients largely ignored.

"So we take Jenny home with us in a few days and all should be fine. Is that what you are saying?" Sara asked as her occupational therapist persona rose to the occasion during our next talk with our Easter Seals rep.

"Yes, that's what we are saying," our therapist answered. "We're always here if it doesn't work out."

We were skeptical but knew we weren't in a position to further challenge the decision. As parents of a child with mental health issues, you quickly learn that a lack of cooperation could result in even fewer services.

Jenny was discharged a few weeks later. The first few days went reasonably well. She returned to the school for kids with behavioral problems and, after about a week, a blowup resulted in a meeting with school teachers and administrators. This time, Jenny had refused to calm herself during one of her escalated states. She'd been told she would have to go to time-out if she didn't quiet herself. She refused and staff were forced to physically restrain her to get her into the time-out room. During the scuffling, she swung one of her arms and struck a teacher's aide. The result was that Jenny stayed home for a couple of days before returning to school.

Things were going about the same at home as they were at school. Jenny's oppositional behavior had resumed and on occasion, she would say very nasty things to her mother. Sara's mental capacity and quickness had diminished over the course of the past eighteen months and Jenny, always able to find and take advantage of a weakness, discovered she could inflict mental and emotional pain and anguish on Sara by calling her names, making fun of her, or picking up on her inability to do things she could once do.

I had often likened Jenny, when agitated, to a cornered animal. She would lash out in the most direct and mean ways, doing just about anything she could to help her feel less diminished. The hurtful things that came out of her mouth often struck very hard. It usually took all the focus and restraint we could muster to stay calm and avoid engaging Jenny in an argument that, sometimes, would become physical, but often resulted in Sara leaving the room. I would usually find her later, crying in our bedroom.

"Why does she have to be so nasty and mean?" Sara would ask rhetorically. "I have worked with kids like this for years and I can't remember one who was so nasty."

I took Sara in my arms and reminded her that this was very different than what she had experienced with her patients. Jenny was our child and that, coupled with Sara's advanced stage of illness, made it an altogether different situation.

"I know," Sara said in response to my comments, choking back her tears, "but why does she have to be this way? I don't understand."

I looked into her tearful eyes and responded. "I don't know why she is this way, but I do know that all we can do is keep working at this and try to make it better. I really do believe it'll end up working out. With that said, we both know how difficult it is to get verbally assaulted as we do. We just have to keep at it."

Sara nodded but didn't respond. She already knew the reality of what I was saying and fully understood. We had discussed it on many previous occasions. We knew, and had accepted, hanging in and doing what we could for Jenny was our only real alternative.

As the next few weeks passed, we found our interactions with Jenny reverting to the level we had experienced prior to her being institutionalized. With increasing frequency, our phones were connected to our therapists. Not surprisingly, they said there wasn't much they could do as far as returning Jenny to in-patient treatment was concerned.

Jenny's prediction had become reality. As she had said, she wasn't ready for this. And at times it seemed she was driven to prove she was right.

Yet another discussion with our Easter Seals therapist gave us hope they had a solution, and a couple of days later, after dropping Jenny at school, we went to meet with Shari.

"I know you've been having difficult times," she said. "We've been talking about Jenny and have considered several options. We believe the best solution at this time is to place her in foster care."

Sara and I looked at one another. We were a bit confused at the suggestion and voiced that as we talked further.

"I understand your concerns and would expect you to have questions. In the end, though, we're prepared to make this work for you, and for Jenny. We want to see how she can adapt to another family situation as she makes more progress," she said as we prepared to leave.

Sara and I were unsure about this. We thought about Jenny being in another family dynamic and wondered how that would help her behave more appropriately. However, we knew we had limited options. One thing was certain: it wasn't working as things were.

As we expected, explaining this new direction was not easy. Shari joined us as we attempted to help Jenny make sense of it all.

"I don't understand why I can't stay with Mom and Dad," she said to our therapist. "Things are better now than they used to be. And I'll be better. I promise."

If only it were that easy, I thought as I listened to Jenny's pleas. In the end, Sara and I had very mixed feelings as Shari took her off to her foster family.

There was consternation, but also relief, as the two of them left. We had gotten very used to, and comfortable with, being in a place without bickering, arguing, or physical confrontation. Jenny's return had escalated the stress level in the house.

After a few days, we had a conversation with Shari about visiting Jenny. We waited a day before driving past the home in Pontiac, one of the rougher Detroit suburbs. A couple of days later, we arranged to stop and see how she was doing. Jenny not only had to adjust to her foster parents, but also to the six other foster children in the home. She seemed okay and we left after about an hour. Sara cried as we drove away.

"I'm so torn," she said between sobs. "Those people seem nice and mean well and I don't think it is a bad thing Jenny is around some other kids. But she seemed distant and out of place."

"I know," I answered, acknowledging that Jenny seemed confused and a bit withdrawn. "But we have to have some trust in Easter Seals. They've been good to us. We should give it some time to see if it helps her."

A few days later, we were able to take Jenny for a couple of hours and we talked about her placement.

"It's okay, I guess," she said. "The other kids are nice and I like being around most of them."

She grew quiet as we drove toward Troy and then asked another question.

"I don't understand. Is the family in Pontiac my real family, or are they just my family until Easter Seals finds someone else? Are you guys still my family? I want to be with you, Andrew, Murphy, and Allie."

Sara worked hard to hold back her tears and I attempted to answer Jenny's questions.

"Jen," I said, "we are always family. You, me, Mom, Andrew, the dogs. We're always your family. I think the best way for you to look at this is that they are your temporary family and are trying to help you learn to behave better so you can live with us again."

Sara had composed herself and chimed in. "Jenny, you are our little girl and always will be. As we have often said, you have to be able to manage yourself. If you can't, then someone else, like the police or therapists, have to. If they can't manage you, then you've got to go someplace that can manage you—like CHD or this foster home. Like always, we want you at home with us and hope that will happen soon."

Jenny grew quiet, then asked, "How long before we're home? I can't wait to see Murphy."

We soon arrived at home and Jenny did a quick walk-through of the house, carrying Murphy with her as she did. She then went up to her room, where she stayed for most of her visit.

Later the following week, we learned that the teacher's aide Jenny had struck, as staff tried to place her in time-out a few weeks earlier, had filed an assault charge with the police. It meant Jenny would have to face the court in Oakland County.

Over the next several weeks, Jenny seemed to make a bit of progress. Also, Jenny's court date had been set and we prepared for our visit with a judge.

Our Easter Seals representative and the foster mom joined us for the court date. On hand, too, was the police officer who answered the complaint. Jenny sat very still as the judge explained the charges brought against her. As the judge continued talking, Jenny suddenly smirked and quietly laughed about something.

"Jenny, is there something funny about your being here, in front of this court?" the judge asked, obviously not amused with Jenny's attitude.

Jenny seemed to understand the severity of the matter and sat up straight and got quiet.

"No," she replied, looking down at her lap.

"You need to understand something, Jenny," added the representative of the court, a stern tone in her voice. "The charge brought against you is very serious. You need to take it that way. If you choose not to, you are making a big mistake. Do you understand?"

Jenny quietly said yes.

The judge asked the police officer for his testimony and he matter-of-factly went through the details of the incident. The judge then asked to hear Jenny's side of the story, which she recounted. Shari offered statements about Jenny and how Easter Seals had been working with her for a long time. She also explained our family situation. It was obvious the judge had not known of Sara's illness. The foster mom also provided some nice comments about Jenny.

The judge again turned to Jenny and asked her what she had to say about the matter.

"I didn't mean to hit anyone," Jenny said. "I just didn't want to go into time-out. I was trying to keep them from picking me up and my arm hit her. It was an accident."

The judge took a few minutes to consider what she had heard.

"Jenny" she said, "when I first read about what you did and I looked at your history, I was prepared to place you in a juvenile facility. But after hearing what your social worker, your foster mother, and your parents have to say, I'm going to recommend something else. You must start seriously looking at your behavior and change it. I want you to write, every day, about how you're working to change it and then send me what you write. You must keep up in your school work, not get into any further trouble, and focus on doing what you must to improve how you interact with your parents and others. If you can do that, you'll be absolved of this charge. If not, you will be placed in the juvenile home. Do you understand?"

The mention of "juvey" had gotten Jenny's attention. It was a place she had frequently talked about in a negative way. She was always adamant about not going and cried at the mention of it.

"Yes, I understand," she said, sobbing. "I promise to do all those things and I'll do better. I promise."

The judge closed the proceedings by reiterating to Jenny that her behavior must change or there would be severe consequences.

We quietly left the courthouse. Jenny had little to say as we drove her back to the foster home. She gave us both big hugs as we left and said how she would do better.

Things seemed to improve over the next couple of months, but an incident with the other foster children—one that was not of Jenny's making—brought the whole thing down. After Easter Seals looked into it, they decided Jenny had to be moved elsewhere.

She was placed in another foster home in early August. It was a far different environment, a home on several acres in rural Oakland County. It seemed almost idyllic, and Jenny appeared to embrace the change.

After talking with our social worker, we had some concerns. We sensed she did as well. The mother, the point person in running the home, had just completed training that qualified her to deal with kids with severe behavioral and emotional challenges. We wondered if she was truly prepared to deal with an adolescent with an illness, and behavior, as severe as Jenny's.

Jenny moved into the home and when we visited, she really seemed to like it. As we learned more, we discovered that the other kids in the house had quickly become afraid of Jenny. Further, the foster mother had told Easter Seals that Jenny intimidated her.

On a late August Friday, we picked up Jenny for the weekend and were looking forward to having her home. The mood quickly changed as we left. Jenny seemed agitated. I hadn't driven five minutes before she challenged Sara and me on some minor point and began to argue. She continued to escalate until she was pretty much out of control. I even stopped the car once to make certain the child locks were on so she couldn't jump out.

I called Easter Seals as we neared our home to let them know we were having a particularly difficult time and that I didn't think Jenny could stay for the weekend. Jenny overheard my conversation and demanded that she talk to the person from Easter Seals. I asked the woman on the other end if she was okay with it. She said she was, so I handed the phone to Jenny.

Jenny immediately started yelling at the Easter Seals woman. In the meantime, we had arrived at home and Jenny stayed on the phone, being disrespectful and angry. She went out on our deck so we could not hear her conversation and soon came storming back in the house, yelling and swearing. She threw down the phone, tossed around some items, and smashed a few other things in our family room. She then ran up the stairs and slammed the door to her room.

I picked up the phone and discovered the Easter Seals rep still there. I told her what had transpired and she immediately asked what we planned to do.

"I'm calling the police," I said, trying to remain calm. "Jenny is out of control and knows she cannot behave like this. When she does, others intervene."

Sara had tried to help with the situation, but with Jenny this agitated, she could only retreat, if for no reason other than her own safety.

The Troy police arrived in a few minutes and I explained what had gone on. The officer looked around at the broken items, took a few notes, and then said, "You know, I've been here before. Your daughter's a little Asian girl, right?"

I admitted that this was not our first encounter with Troy's finest.

One of his fellow officers arrived soon thereafter and she questioned me for a few minutes while the other officer went upstairs to speak with Jenny. A few minutes later, he returned and the female officer went upstairs. She came back down after about five minutes and said Jenny had calmed down.

I spoke with the two of them as Sara listened. She had been quiet as the entire matter played out. The officers wanted Jenny evaluated at a hospital and were prepared to call Troy Beaumont when I stopped them.

"We've been through this more than once," I said. "We'll go over there, Jenny will be evaluated, and they'll end up wanting to send her to a psychiatric facility for more evaluation. Jenny was an inpatient at Kingswood Hospital on Eight Mile Road before her last long-term placement. They know us, know her, and have her records. Could the ambulance just transport her there?"

The officers looked at one another and said that sounded reasonable. We waited a few minutes and an ambulance quietly arrived. The attendant went to get Jenny and I heard them chatting and laughing. Jenny spoke as they came down the stairs.

"Hey, Mom and Dad? This guy took me to the hospital the last time I went in," she said as if she was going off for some evening out, a big smile coming over her face.

He said something else to her and they laughed as he took her to the waiting unit. The mood swings of bipolar disorder never ceased to amaze us. We met up with the two of them again when we arrived at Kingswood.

Jenny's intake took a while. There were two others being admitted. Jenny was generally cooperative and calm as the entire process played out and, a few hours later, Sara and I were back home.

I went into the family room and picked up the shattered glass and picture frame that Jenny had broken in her tirade. I searched for other items that were destroyed and tossed them out. At least, I thought, it isn't like the time she got so wound up that she kicked a six-inch hole in the foyer drywall.

It had been a long and exasperating late afternoon and evening. Sara and I were both drained. The dark circles I saw so often under Sara's eyes during her cancer treatments had returned.

"Well, we're back to where Jenny said she should be," she said, recalling what Jenny said nine months earlier. "Sometimes, I think she just wants to show us so she can say 'I told you so.'"

We finished cleaning up the house and went upstairs to bed. Sara crawled in beside me and gave me a big hug.

"I just want to see her make some real progress before I'm not around anymore," she said. "With the right meds and therapy, she has a chance. But she has to want it, too. For some reason, she isn't ready for it yet."

I wondered about the reality of Jenny making real progress.

Jenny's stay at Kingswood didn't last as long as her first. A couple of weeks passed and she was placed at a mental health facility in Auburn Hills called Havenwyck. Jenny had been there on another occasion for short-term treatment and hadn't found it to her liking. She thought they were too strict and even, sometimes, mean.

We reminded her that this was one of those times when she had to be in a place where others managed her because she couldn't manage herself.

Jenny looked at us and started to cry. "I just want to be with the two of you."

As it turned out, Jenny wasn't the only female in my life that was difficult. Sara was starting to show signs of personality changes caused by her brain tumor. She was often distracted and distant. Occasionally, she became very argumentative and oppositional. Sometimes she seemed obsessed with religion and, occasionally, would tell me she had been talking with God.

Sara's commitment to her Lutheran faith had always been strong. On the occasions when we moved, one of the first things she did was find a church. We had frequently talked about it and agreed that the basic Christian values that came with belonging to a Lutheran church were good for the kids. We sometimes didn't agree when she moved down the literal Biblical path. While she generally accepted Lutheran doctrine, I was far more skeptical and often didn't agree with church positions. That said, I had decided I would bite my tongue and "go along to get along" as we dealt with matters religious.

I found it troubling that Sara was becoming more immersed in the church. It seemed to be a reflection of her need to place her illness in God's hands. While I am spiritual, I generally find the hypocrisy, politics, backbiting, and infighting within church organizations to be at odds with spiritual needs. It made it difficult, at times, for me to support Sara's interest in our church.

Sara used our church for many of her relationships. While she remained closest to her friend Marilyn, she was growing extremely well connected to the church. It concerned me in that we had always looked at our church affiliation as part of a balanced approach to our lives. Sara's interest in placing the church front and center in her life was taking precedence, and the balance we had worked hard to cultivate and maintain was diminishing.

I brought it up late in 2003 and wished I had not done so as soon as I'd spoken. I told her I thought she was putting too much emphasis on the church and God's place in our life.

"Ron, how can you say that?" she said, a genuine sense of hurt in her voice. "Jesus guides us through our lives and shows us the way."

I was not interested in discussing the virtues of the Christian faith and told her I didn't think it was healthy for us to be so narrowly devoted to any one belief. She immediately became quiet, and I knew this was a discussion that was only going to drive a wedge between us. I was reminded of the old adage, "There are three things to avoid in conversation: religion, sex, and politics." I just never thought any of that would apply to our relationship. Sara and I had spent countless hours over the years openly and honestly discussing these topics. It had always been enjoyable. We disagreed at times but generally came to the same conclusions. That was changing with Sara's more single-minded thinking, and it was a loss I felt deeply. It further confirmed the personality change I was seeing in her. I was saddened to think I was losing yet another piece of her.

As the year wound down, Andrew was well into his junior year at Western Michigan, and Jenny continued her stay at Havenwyck, struggling to reach some level of normalcy. My fledgling business as a financial representative was just a few months old and trying to get its footing.

I sometimes wondered about the stress that dealing with a mentally ill child brought into our lives. Countless research studies show a real relationship between stress and illness. Sara's cancer first appeared in 1983 and Jenny became part of the family in 1988. I sometimes wondered if it had affected the progression of Sara's illness.

Then, too, I had experienced my bout with cancer in 2000. Neither Sara nor I had any reason to believe we would have the disease. There were no real traces of it in our family histories and no known exposure to any external influences that would bring on such an outcome.

Could it have been driven by the stress we experienced in trying to manage Jenny? It was a question we never would, or could, answer. But it was natural to speculate.

I also wondered about how stress impacted me in a more general sense. When we first started experiencing the episodes with Jenny, I regularly reacted in a way that could be pretty intense. Anger about her name-calling and physical opposition was not unusual. There was never any physical abuse, but I sometimes used some strong words. Sara and I would often tag team the situation, restraining Jenny when necessary while trying to bring her down from the manic moments she experienced.

As we navigated a heavy-duty regime of family therapy, we began to understand our feelings and learned strategies and tactics that allowed us to more effectively deal with Jenny's outbursts. Key lessons learned included: the importance of staying calm and not overwhelming her with too much information; accepting that our parenting had nothing to do with her outbursts; and understanding that use of physical restraint, properly applied, was all right in certain circumstances. Often, they were tough lessons to process, but it was imperative to learn them if we were to survive this and carry on.

The therapy was critical to managing all that I had coming at me. I would sometimes sit after Sara went to bed and wonder why. Why had she become ill? Where would it all end up? How did she get breast cancer? Could we have done anything differently to change the result? Was I doing enough to take care of myself as I dealt with it?

I went through the various stages: the disbelief, anger, sadness and, ultimately, acceptance of what we faced. I sat through dozens of therapy sessions and came to understand just how valuable they were. Therapy was a terrific resource for me, one that allowed me to vent, to openly and honestly express my feelings about a life turned upside down. I learned all this was okay.

But I fairly quickly came to understand the necessity of carrying on—the need to deal with what we faced in an even-keeled, yet focused, manner. I often felt detached and situations seemed surreal as our life unfolded and we moved forward.

But I found there was little time for that thinking. And in the end, it served no real benefit. Sara and I would soon be faced with some major decisions as the calendar turned to 2004. It would be a turning point year for us.

Sara's condition was worsening by the week. Her personality continued to change. She would get short at times—sometimes quite angry—and then would fall back to being the woman I had known for most of my adult life. I was never quite sure who I would encounter as the day began. There were also times when the tumor in her head would push more directly on the tissue around her brain stem and she would go on a round of steroid treatments to reduce the swelling.

The steroids seemed to have a profound effect on Sara, and she would regularly go with little or no sleep as they coursed through her body. As hours became days, she would become agitated and, at times, unwilling to cooperate as I tried to care for her. She sometimes became nasty in her tone and tenor and, while I understood she was experiencing changes in her brain, it didn't lessen the hurt and discouragement I felt in those moments when she lashed out. It was a very difficult time for me, as her caregiver. And it was sometimes difficult not to be pulled down.

In January, she went on yet another round of steroids. I would awaken in the middle of the night to find her in our office downstairs, watching religious television channels or scribbling notes that, upon examination, made little, if any, sense. As the steroids tapered off, she would come back to a state somewhat more normal, and we would go along for a few weeks before the episode repeated itself.

In early February, Dr. Decker and his team let us know that the neurosurgeon who had considered surgery several months before was again examining her case. They understood the need to try to do more to help Sara at this stage of her illness. The doctor had consulted with his Beaumont colleagues and had also reached out to physicians from the cancer and neurology units at Henry Ford Hospital.

As they went through Sara's case, they came to the conclusion that she had reached a place where she was a good candidate for surgery. After hearing from the neurology team, Dr. Decker informed us that he was thinking that a surgical procedure to remove the tumor could be a success. He suggested we meet with the neurosurgeon.

We met with the surgeon and he was optimistic that the surgery would improve Sara's life.

"We've had some of the best neurosurgeons around look through your films and discuss your case," he said. "We've come to the conclusion that the tumor has increased in size to the point that we can now remove it with minimal risk of damage to adjacent tissue. That said, there is always a risk when you do surgery and, while we want to do all we can to minimize the risk, the reality is that there is still a risk."

Sara and I listened intently and silence filled the room when he finished speaking.

"So, what do you think?" he said, breaking the silence.

Sara and I looked at one another and didn't hesitate. We knew we were running out of options and this was one of the few we had left.

"I think I want to try it," Sara said. "I have very little to lose; lots to gain if it works."

I was hesitant. Even though the doctor had been open with us about the surgery, I knew the risks were not small. I also knew Sara's quality of life could be diminished greatly if it did not go the way we hoped.

"We should think about this," I offered. I knew Sara was ready and, for the most part, I was, too. It was just that this was a big-time decision, one that would impact our lives dramatically, regardless of the outcome.

"Except for not surviving the surgery, what would be the worst-case outcome in this scenario?" I asked, wondering how forthright the doctor would be in his response.

"This procedure is in a very delicate section of the brain," he said. "If the surgery goes the way it should, there will be no damage to adjacent tissue. I would not be truthful with you, though, if I said this is not a challenging surgery. It is. It will go on for several hours and, as I said, there is always a risk. That risk could include reduced or lost ability of an autonomic function—such as seeing, breathing, smelling or tasting. I wish I could offer a guarantee, but I can't."

We continued our conversation in the car. Sara was excited about the potential. If nothing else, it signified doing something. We each felt we had, at best, been treading water over the past year. Sara had continued her Herceptin and Zometa treatments, but we understood them to be little more than maintenance. This surgery brought some hope, however small it might be. We talked a bit more about it that evening, and the next morning, Sara called to say that she was ready to move ahead with the surgery. The doctor's scheduler called back soon after and the operation was set for early in April.

I saw a real change in Sara's behavior as the next few weeks unfolded. When we were with friends, she enthusiastically told them of her pending procedure. When they asked about the complexity and risks associated with it—as they inevitably did—Sara responded in an almost dismissive manner.

"This'll be a breeze," she said one evening when we were at church, at one of the ever-popular Lutheran potluck dinners, sitting around a big table with several friends.

"I don't expect I'll be in the hospital more than a couple of days. We're ready for it, and when it is complete and I come through it all, I'll be good for several more years."

Those sitting at the table appeared uncomfortable as they listened. They looked away or down at the table as Sara spoke. They sensed the seriousness of the surgery. In her unending efforts to project a positive perspective, Sara was demonstrating how her cognitive functioning had changed and diminished, and it minimized her credibility among her friends.

I did, however, admire her courage and resolve, especially since I knew the reality of the procedure. I never came to a place where I fully understood how much she believed about the things she said as she prepared for the procedure. But she continued to say them and I didn't question them. I figured that with her never-ending focus on being the best patient she could be, she needed to say what she did, even if she was saying it to convince herself that the operation was the right thing to do.

It was further indication of her willingness to do what she could to continue to fight the disease. Underneath it all, I believe she knew how challenging the surgery would be. But she would never admit it to anyone. And especially not to herself.

We had moved to that place we didn't ever want to be: the disease was dictating our decisions. Sure, we could do nothing, but that choice left us staring at an inevitability we certainly understood—and did not want.

As Sara was doing, I had to come to accept the realities of the surgery and was prepared to make the best of it.

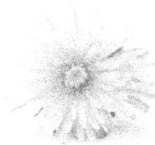

CHAPTER

14

The early April surgery day came sooner than we wanted. Sara was on steroids the final days before the surgery and was energized. As generally was the case when she was on the drug, her behavior turned odd, even bizarre, at times. She often referenced how God was taking care of us and that she had talked with him. She continued, and sometimes increased, her unrealistically optimistic talk about how she would rebound from the surgery. She also became quite amorous—an unexpected and surprising change—and told me it would be that way all the time following the surgery.

I smiled and pulled her close as we savored the moments following a round of "afternoon delight."

"I know and that will be great," I said, humoring her, as we hugged and traded kisses. "And that was pretty good for a couple of old folks."

Silence returned as the reality of our lives washed back over us. Sara spoke up a couple minutes later.

"I'm really looking forward to having this surgery, having this tumor removed from my brain. I have total faith in my doctors and their abilities. God has given them extraordinary talent and I know he will make sure this all goes well."

I felt my discomfort level rise and wanted to change the direction of the discussion.

"We really have been fortunate to find such great doctors," I said. "I know they are confident this will go well, and I think so, too."

The feelings underlying my comment were less certain than those Sara expressed. Since making the decision to proceed, I had thought many times of the risks. My mind frequently wondered about the outcome. Fear of that unknown was a constant.

Andrew and Jenny joined us to go to Beaumont very early, and I sat with Sara as she was prepped for the surgery. She had shaved her head the night before, giving her the look she had sported during her chemo days, and she had broken out the scarves and caps that had become daily accessories during those times. We joked about it as she went through them. I acted as if they needed to be dusted off and started a manufactured cough as she dug through the container that housed them.

The pre-op area was bustling. Nurses darted around, reviewing charts, going over disclosure forms and getting final signatures, starting IVs, and offering cheery presurgical support. Andrew and Jenny spent some of the time with us, and I convinced them to go get some breakfast at the Beaumont cafeteria since all three of us would not be allowed to stay with Sara in the pre-op area. The anesthesiologist came by and briefed us on his piece of the plan. Then Sara's surgeon came into the curtained space.

"Are we ready for what lies ahead?" he asked.

"We're ready," Sara said, the smile on her face bubbling up in her voice. "I can't wait to get this over with and get on with life."

"We—the entire surgical team—are ready, too," he said with a smile. "Do you have any questions?"

We had no questions; we were ready. The curtain slid closed behind him and Sara and I were alone. I squeezed her hand tightly as we looked at one another. I asked if she was okay and she assured me she was ready and that all would go fine.

"I love you," she said as the curtain slid open and a nurse appeared.

"We're ready for you, Sara," she said.

An orderly pulled the side rails up on the gurney and I reluctantly let go of Sara's hand. I stood and leaned over the rail to give her a kiss.

"I'll see you in a little while," I said. "I love you."

She smiled at me and mouthed "I love you, too," as the gurney rolled away.

I left the pre-op area and went to find Andrew and Jenny. It would be a long day.

We spent the rest of the morning in the waiting area adjacent to a large and beautiful atrium. As I settled into an overstuffed, leather chair, I thought of the dozens of other times I had waited in hospitals and other healthcare facilities in Denver, Milwaukee, and here. It was unusual to have such a beautiful space available for families and loved ones.

Several small trees and a variety of other plants thrived in the spacious atrium. The Michigan springtime sunshine made a welcome appearance, warming the area. Its brilliance was almost blinding on this April day.

The surgery started around 8:15 and a nurse from the surgical team came by soon after to let us know they had begun. The surgeon, she said, figured the procedure would last about four to five hours. The nurse was a frequent visitor as the day progressed, and it was good to know we were being kept abreast of what was happening.

We were about to head to lunch when I saw her coming down the hallway.

"I'm glad I caught you. I wanted to give you an update," she said. "All is going well, but a bit more slowly than we expected. It looks like the surgery will probably go longer than anticipated. I will let you know more when I know more."

Jenny asked me if everything was all right with Mom.

"I think so," I said. "We can't forget how delicate this surgery is. They're working in Mom's brain so they have to be very careful. If that means taking more time to do it than they originally thought, that's okay."

We returned to the atrium after lunch and waited. And waited. About 2:30, the nurse reappeared and said they were getting close to finishing. The surgical team expected it would be another hour. True to form, about 3:30 she returned and said the surgery was complete and that the doctor would soon be out to speak with us.

Sara's surgeon soon came down the hallway and sat down. He looked exhausted.

"Everything went well," he said with a weak smile. "Sara is in recovery and doing fine. You will be able to see her before long. As you know, it took longer than we expected. But we wanted to make sure we were extremely careful to minimize the potential for any complications."

I looked hard into his tired face, trying to read past his words. I wondered how well he and his team had truly done in avoiding those complications.

"So, did you get the entire tumor?" I asked.

He paused before he spoke, and I sensed he was being careful in what he said.

"In the area where we were working, it is extremely sensitive," he said. "We believe we got all of the tumor and we took a reasonable margin of adjacent tissue. I don't expect there will be any long-term complications, but we noticed that she has a problem with swallowing. Her epiglottis is not closing at quite the right time when she swallows, and she aspirates slightly each time she swallows. I don't think it will be long-term. Overall, the surgery went extremely well. She tolerated being under anesthesia for a long period very well."

He told us we would be able to go to the ICU and see her soon and reiterated his confidence that all would be well. I thanked him and turned to the kids and our friend, Marilyn, who had joined us. They had heard parts of what the doctor said and looked to me for reaction.

"It sounds like it went well," I said, remaining as positive as possible. "Let's go see her and then we'll have to wait to see how things go."

We boarded the elevator and took it to the floor that housed the ICU. The nurse behind the desk smiled and asked if we were there to see Sara.

"She just started coming around from her anesthesia, but is very groggy," she said. "Let us get her vitals and make sure she is awake enough to have you visit."

We could see through the window behind the desk that one of the nurse's colleagues was with Sara, taking her blood pressure and checking other vital signs. We went to a small waiting area and sat for a few minutes until the nurse gave us the go-ahead.

I slowly opened the door and looked at Sara as we approached the bed. It was raised to about a forty-five degree angle and Sara was propped up, her eyes closed. Her head was wrapped in a winding trail of white gauze and a tube ran out of the bandages and down the back of her neck to a small bag. The beeping of monitors was the lone sound in the room as we quietly approached her bed.

I touched her right thigh as I got close and, in a quiet voice said, "Sara?"

She slowly opened her eyes and the kids moved in alongside the bed, Andrew on the opposite side and Jenny standing to my right.

"Sara? How are you doing?" I asked.

Her eyes opened as she tried to shrug off the anesthesia's effects.

"Hi guys," she said softly.

Her eyes again closed. It was obvious this would be a short visit because she was drifting in and out of consciousness.

I turned to the kids to say that we probably should stay just a few minutes. I had mindlessly started to rub Sara's right thigh as I stood there, not really aware of what I was doing. Suddenly, she came to and admonished me.

"I'm not a dog!" she said. "Stop rubbing my leg!"

I was startled by her response and looked at Andrew. There was a pause and a brief silence before the three of us laughed quietly.

"I'm sorry; I'll stop," I said, smiling at her as her eyes closed and she again nodded off.

We stayed a few more minutes and then left the room. I told the nurse at the station that I would be back later. We headed to the parking lot. I wanted the kids to get away from the tension of the hospital, and Marilyn would drive them home. I suggested they get something to eat with Marilyn and spend some time at home trying to relax a little. I stayed at the hospital until I could see Sara again, just before I left for the evening.

As I was driving home, I wondered just how the issue with her swallowing would turn out. I had no reason to think it was not going to improve, but there was a nagging feeling about it that created a knot in my stomach.

The kids were anxious to hear more about their mom's recovery when I got home. I told them she was mainly sleeping and had spent very little time knowing I was in the room. Marilyn had stayed with the kids while I was at the hospital, and I thanked her for her support throughout the day. After she left, we sat down together in the family room. The television was on but no one was really watching it.

Andrew asked if his mom was going to be okay and whether the issue with her swallowing was going to be a problem. Jenny moved forward, poised to hear what I was going to say about it. Clearly, they were both concerned.

I honestly told them that I didn't know and we would have to wait and see. I assured them that we just needed to be patient and help her as much as we could while she recovered. She would be fine.

But, of course, I couldn't be sure that she would be fine.

"Mom will be all right, won't she?" Jenny asked as I tucked her in.

"I think she will, Jen," I said. "All we can do now is pray for her to fully recover." I pulled the comforter up to her chin and leaned in to kiss her forehead. "Let's just think good thoughts about this. That's what your mom would want and what she is doing. Get some sleep so you can go back to see her again tomorrow. We'll go see her in the morning and then I'll take you back to Havenwyck."

"Can't I stay here until mom comes home? she asked. "Please . . ."

I was firm with Jenny, reminding her that we had agreed she could be there for the surgery but she would have to return to the psych facility after that.

She reluctantly said she understood and would go back, even if she didn't want to.

Andrew was preparing for bed in his room across the hall as I closed his sister's door.

"Is Mom really going to be okay?" he asked, echoing Jenny's concerns.

I hesitated for a moment before I answered. "I don't know, Andrew. None of us—including the doctors—do. They think they got all of the tumor and they don't expect her swallowing issues to continue. I think she'll be fine, but we'll just have to wait to see."

There was little else to say. We were wiped out from the long day. I went to our room to get ready for bed. The dogs had gone out for their final pit stop and were ready for bed, too. Allie went in with Andrew and Murphy with Jenny.

I felt very alone as I crawled into bed, searching for comfort in my thoughts. Neither reading nor television could hold my concentration. I finally surrendered to sleep, wondering what I would find when I went back to Beaumont in a few hours.

All three of us went to see Sara the following morning. Andrew was planning on returning to Kalamazoo later that day and Jenny needed to return to the psychiatric facility, but it was a comfort that we had time that morning to spend as a family with her. And we all needed that. Upon arrival, we found that Sara was about to be moved from the ICU to a semiprivate room. We waited as they prepared to move her and then caravanned to her room where we gathered around her bed.

Sara was more with it but still drifting in and out. She was doing remarkably well, considering she had been in surgery for seven hours the previous day. What wasn't getting better was her swallowing function. Each time she took a drink of water or tried a bite of Jell-O, a portion ended up going down the wrong pipe and into her lungs. It was worrisome because aside from causing violent coughing spells, it also increased her risk for contracting pneumonia. We spent the rest of the morning with her, amid various doctor visits, tests, and scans, before I took Andrew to the train station and Jenny back to the psych facility she'd called home for the past seven months.

When I returned to the hospital and asked Sara how she was doing, she stared at me and said dryly, "I have a headache."

I laughed and said, "Well, I guess you are entitled to one or two of those."

She looked at me for a moment, then realized the humor in it and weakly laughed.

Much later, when I was back home and preparing for bed, the loneliness I'd felt the previous evening washed over me and I sat down on the edge of the bed, staring blankly at the television. Tears formed in my eyes as I thought about where we went from here. I cried quietly for several minutes with the dogs staring at me, as if they sensed my despair and wanted to help. The cry served me well, though, helping me relax.

Suddenly, the phone rang and I immediately thought it might be the hospital with some news. Instead, it was my mother, checking in to see how Sara was doing. Since my father's death in 2002, I made of point of noting where she was on the "lonely meter" when we talked, and her loneliness seeped through the phone as we talked. I was too exhausted and lonely, myself, to be of much comfort to her.

I put Murphy on the end of the bed, something we allowed only occasionally, and Allie jumped up into bed with me. Being more than sixty pounds, she took up a good amount of space on the bed. We usually didn't allow it, in part because she shed her wiry, yellow lab fur. But I had so little energy, I didn't even try to move her. Plus, there was a sense of mutual comforting between me and the dogs. I quickly nodded off.

I remained hopeful Sara's swallowing would return to normal. It weighed heavily on my mind as I returned the following day to Beaumont's cancer unit.

I was disappointed to find there was no change. She was taking her nutrition through an intravenous line as had been the case the previous two days. Each time she tried swallowing something—even saliva—a portion of it traveled into her lungs. She often coughed for extended periods. It sapped her energy and she was beginning to become frustrated. We worried constantly about pneumonia.

She had started light physical and occupational therapy sessions in her room and seemed in decent spirits. But the concern about her swallowing never diminished.

I spent the day with her, responding to a few calls from my financial clients. As darkness settled in, I headed home and found myself dealing, again, with the profound sense of loneliness that had overcome me the last couple of evenings. It was a new feeling for me and I was puzzled about why it now was manifesting itself.

The truth was that I had felt a growing sense of loss and distance from Sara over the past few months. It was easy to dismiss since I was busy with caring for her and doing what I could to make a few dollars as a financial rep. But it was a growing concern and something I recognized as a problem that I was going to have to deal with. It had to wait, though. I didn't have time to address it now.

Sara's inability to swallow normally continued to be a problem. I had talked with her doctors about what would happen if her swallowing function did not soon return. The reality was that none of us wanted to go there. A PEG (Percutaneous Endoscopic Gastrostomy) tube—essentially a feeding tube—was mentioned as a temporary solution to allow Sara to get something in her stomach. The food would come in the form of liquids but the tube would be a better alternative than having IVs deliver nutrients to her.

When I was completely honest with myself, I had to admit I had serious doubts about Sara's chances of regaining the ability to swallow. My intuition said that her doctors were quite unsure about what would happen. For the short term, I was willing to give it the benefit of the doubt. Maybe it was me trying to stay positive, but we had to give it a chance.

Beyond the problems with her swallowing, I had noticed that Sara was losing some of her mental capacity. Her personality didn't seem to be affected in any major way but her ability to deal with and manage numbers, for instance, was not the same. She often was confused about the day, date, and time and it worried me.

Beginning with the week to come, her doctors had prescribed more intense physical, occupational, and speech therapy sessions. She would stay at the hospital, they said, at least through the next week to do her therapy, as well as keep an eye on her recovery.

But we had to deal with the immediate problem: her ability to ingest food. Sara's doctor and his colleagues had discussed her progress and felt it important that Sara get off the IVs. He explained they wanted to implant the PEG tube. A short surgery put the tube in place.

"I was afraid it might come down to this," she said, her normally positive demeanor slipping away. She examined the tubing that was taped to the lower portion of her stomach and went silent for a few moments before she continued. "I don't want you doing my feedings. I'll do them."

I nodded my understanding and sensed her frustration with the process. The familiar feeling of loss hit me as I stood at her bedside. As always, we would do what we needed to do.

The idea of eating through a tube had little appeal to Sara. Several times she had voiced her desire to eat real food, even if it was hospital food—and this was a blow to her confidence. She needed to learn how to properly use the tube and reluctantly agreed to have a nurse walk her through the process.

The nurse returned a bit later with a can of liquid similar to Ensure and a large syringe without a needle or plunger. She removed the tape holding the end of the tube against Sara's stomach and inserted the nose of the syringe into the tube's opening. She had opened the can and it was sitting on the hospital tray next to the bed.

Sara watched intently as the nurse did her preparations. She asked a couple of questions as the nurse held the top of the syringe about six inches above Sara's abdomen and slowly poured the thick, beige liquid into the device's tube. It filled, then began to drain into Sara's stomach. The nurse refilled the syringe and, again, it slowly drained. Sara said she could feel the thick liquid running into her stomach, and she almost immediately started to belch.

"It's weird. I can taste it even though I didn't drink it," she said.

"That's something I often hear when we do this," the nurse replied. "It's important we get your system working again, to have some food in your stomach."

I had watched with great interest, knowing, despite Sara's wishes, that I would be doing this in the near future.

The nurse continued the feeding and concluded in about five minutes. Sara continued to occasionally belch and voiced her displeasure with the taste she had in her mouth.

"Well, even if it was liquid out of a can, it is something in your stomach," I said as Sara made a face to convey her dislike of the taste of her first meal in several days.

"I can do this myself," she said of the feeding procedure.

Later in the day, when a nurse came in with another can of liquid, Sara had her first opportunity to practice.

I connected the nose of the syringe to the opening in the tube and then opened the can. Sara held the syringe in her left hand while grasping the can in her right. I watched, a sense of apprehension coming over me. This had to work. If

Sara couldn't do it, her self-confidence would be dealt another blow.

She slowly lifted the can and tried to pour it into the syringe. A small amount went into the tube, but she lost her bearings and the can slipped aside the syringe, the liquid splashing onto her stomach and hospital gown. She pulled the can back and looked at me. I had a good idea where this was going to end but I sat silently, letting her do what she must.

She again lifted the can toward the syringe. Her left hand, which had not been steady on her first attempt, now began to shake more violently as she lifted the can.

I decided it was time to intervene and offered to help.

A look of resignation came over her face as she passed me the can. I moved closer and took the syringe from her left hand. I raised the tube above her stomach as she sat on the side of her bed. I poured the liquid into the syringe and watched it slowly run down the tube and into Sara's stomach. As long as my hand was steady, the process was not difficult. The key was staying on top of how Sara was feeling. She would ask to stop for short periods of time to let the liquid settle in her stomach. I completed the task, closed the tubing, and re-taped it to her stomach. My first attempt to help had been a success.

When I got ready to leave for the day, Sara pulled me close and gave me a bigger than usual hug.

"I love you so much," she said. "Thanks for being here for me."

The reality of this was sinking in for her. We didn't have to talk about it in any greater depth. I knew what her hug meant.

As I headed down the hall and waited for the elevator, I thought about my life. A Saturday evening in the spring. I'm heading home from the hospital at 8:30 p.m., dog tired and ready to go to bed. Not exactly what I'd expected to be doing at this stage of my life. When we walked down the aisle in that Lutheran church in Wauseon in 1975, I figured we would be married at least fifty years, probably longer. Filling a feeding tube in my seriously ill fifty-one-year-old wife's stomach wasn't on that agenda.

As the new week started, Sara spent a good part of her day in physical and occupational therapy. I was a little surprised when she asked me to join her for her sessions the next day. I wondered why she wanted me there and asked her if something was wrong.

"I don't know. I'm feeling it isn't going like it should. I want you to be there to make sure they are doing what they should be doing to help me."

It was out of character for Sara to say something like this. She had always been supportive of her doctors and nurses. I knew she wouldn't question an individual she saw as a colleague unless she had a serious concern. I promised to be there to watch and tell her what I thought.

The next day, I discovered Sara in relatively good spirits and looking forward to her physical therapy. She worked on muscle strength and did some stretching. Her long days in bed had sapped her and her muscles had atrophied. She tired easily and quickly.

After the physical therapy session, she was wheeled by a nurse's aide to the waiting area outside speech therapy. We were soon joined by the speech therapist and Sara introduced me.

The therapist worked on Sara's swallowing function first. It was difficult to watch as a small mirror, similar to a dental instrument, was inserted in Sara's mouth and reached the back of her throat where the speech therapist moved it to facilitate Sara's swallowing. Sara gagged several times, but she didn't back away from the process.

After that, the therapist reached for a manila folder and pulled out a sheet of paper. On it was a small paragraph and a simple map of the Midwest. It was a word problem requiring Sara do basic math to get the answer.

I stood behind her and watched as the therapist asked her to read it aloud.

Sara slowly read the words, "One train is headed west from Chicago going forty-nine miles per hour. A second train leaves Des Moines and is headed east going fifty-five. The distance between the two cities is 332 miles. When and where will the two pass one another?"

Sara struggled as she read the problem. She had always been an avid reader and was proficient at simple math. It was difficult to watch her labor as she was.

"I'd like you to figure out the problem and give me an answer, okay, Sara?" the therapist said.

The speech therapist move to her desk on the other side of the room. Sara looked at the paper on the table. Several minutes went by as she attempted to solve the problem. After a few minutes, the therapist returned and Sara started to cry.

"I know that I need to able to add and subtract, multiply and divide," she said. "But I don't know how to do it." Her crying turning to sobs as she pushed the paper away.

The therapist quickly intervened and was sympathetic to Sara's building frustration.

"It's all right, Sara," she said. "We'll try another time. Don't worry about it."

"I'd like to go back to my room," Sara said with disgust, her hands on the wheelchair's wheels as she attempted to make it move. "I don't want to do this right now, anyway."

I walked behind the nurse's aide as she pushed Sara back to her room. We sat quietly for several minutes before she spoke.

"This is just another thing that I have lost," she said angrily. "I really want things to be normal again. I want to be able to eat. I want to be able to remember all the things I used to be able to do. I want to be out there, enjoying the spring, planting flowers, and working in our yard. It's depressing to live like this."

I let her go on for a couple of minutes before speaking.

"I know this is hard. I wish it was different, too. It has to be so difficult to be losing things in your life as you have over the past few months."

We just sat with that thought for a couple of minutes before I again broke the silence.

"Where is the woman who always says she wants to be the best patient she can be?"

Sara looked hard at me, then her eyes shifted away. After several seconds, she looked back into my eyes.

"I know you're right," she said, "but it doesn't mean I can't be angry about it. I need to. Please just let me be mad. Soon, I'll be that best patient again."

It was time to stay silent.

I left a few minutes later. We faced a long road.

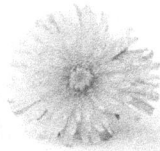

CHAPTER
15

Sara's hospitalization ended up lasting far longer than we expected. After I'd attended her therapy sessions, she remained at Beaumont an additional couple of weeks. She continued her recovery, did her therapy, and finally was discharged near the end of April.

Since she had been gone several weeks, the dogs were excited to see her. I had to keep Allie from pushing her over. Just the brief trip home had worn her down and she wanted to get up the stairs and into bed. Once I helped her get situated, I went downstairs to get some work done.

When it was time for her feeding, I took a break from reviewing client files and mutual fund performance figures and went upstairs. Sara was soundly sleeping and I was hesitant to wake her, but I knew I needed to.

It was a pivotal moment for us. While I had helped feed her several times in the hospital, this was different. We were in our space, not the hospital. Helping her in our own home, in our own kitchen, cemented a feeling of permanence that I hadn't felt in the hospital.

I went to the two cases of liquid nutrition we had sitting in the corner, removed one of the cans, opened it, and sat the large feeding syringe, along with a couple of paper towels, on our kitchen table.

Then I went up to awaken Sara. I thought of the process we were about to experience and wondered if it would end up being temporary, as our doctors continued to insist, or if it would be Sara's plight for the remainder of her life. I pushed the thought to the back of my mind as I roused Sara from her lengthy nap.

"It's already time for me to do my feeding again?" she asked as she slowly awakened.

"Yeah, I have it all ready for you in the kitchen," I said. "Let me help you down the stairs."

We made our way down the steps and I led her to a kitchen chair. I pulled a second seat directly across from her, and sat down, our knees touching. I turned to the table to pick up the syringe and, as I was doing that, Sara pulled her top above her stomach and removed the tape that secured the tube to her.

I looked at the large, "female" end of the tube and my eyes traced back to where it was absorbed by Sara's stomach. I took a deep breath and gently lifted the end of the tubing from her hand. Then I inserted the nose of the syringe in the tube and looked into Sara's eyes. It was a moment that felt very intimate. A closeness we had not experienced in some time fell over us.

"Are you ready?" I asked, grasping her left hand as she held the tube in her right.

Sara hesitated as if she was contemplating the entire process and then offered a weak, "Yes."

I reached for the can, brought it to the space between us and centered it over the syringe. I looked into Sara's eyes and received a visual go-ahead. I slowly tilted the can and the thick liquid began dribbling into the syringe and down the tube. It took a few seconds to run into her stomach.

"I can already taste it. It's so weird," she said. "Honestly, it's awful."

I filled the syringe and watched it slowly draw down into the tube. I repeated the procedure a few more times before the can was empty.

"That's it. That's all of it," I said as the last few drops drained from the can. "Are you doing all right?"

She didn't answer and sat quietly as the tube slowly drained into her stomach. She didn't have to say anything, but I knew as she scanned the kitchen. She was thinking about how many times she had prepared and enjoyed a meal in the very area where we were seated. It had to feel strange for her. I wanted to say something but thought better of bringing it up.

I removed the syringe, went to the sink, rinsed it out, and placed it in the dishwasher. I looked back at Sara and she was pushing the attached flexible closure back into the end of the tube.

"I feel a little sick," she said, belching a few times. "That stuff tastes pretty bad and the smell that comes back up from my stomach makes me a little nauseous."

I tore off a piece of tape and placed the dispenser back in the box. The nurse had been kind enough to stash several roles of tape, as well as a couple of syringes, into a box for our home use. Sara was holding the tube, waiting for me to reapply the tape and attach it to her stomach. When I'd done that, she pulled her top back down and shakily got to her feet.

I asked if she was up to sitting with me for a while. "It seems like such a long time since we have done anything that feels normal."

She forced a weak smile. I knew she would rather be upstairs, but she agreed to stay.

We rounded the half-wall that separated our family room from the kitchen, made our way to the loveseat, and sat down. I fumbled with the television remote and turned on the TV. Both Allie and Murphy were at our feet. Sara picked up the little black-and-white shih tzu and held him like a baby.

"It has been a long time since it *has* felt normal, hasn't it? You know that I understand how difficult this has been for you, too, don't you? I know I've said it before, but I really appreciate all you do, how you are always here for me. You always have been. It means so much."

She looked so tired. I thought of our younger days and the girl I had grown up with. Fallen in love with. It seemed so long ago. I felt my love for her well up inside me. It was a love strong in the way love can only be when two people have shared life's pleasures, but have also navigated through several difficult life-and-death experiences along the way.

We hugged, held one another, and then sat quietly for the next hour or so, the fingers of my left hand laced through the fingers of her right. Sara drifted in and out of sleep while I mindlessly watched the television. Murphy snoozed in her lap and Allie was at my feet.

All was at peace. Normal had returned, even if it was for only a brief few moments.

Sara continued her recovery and her strength returned in very small increments. She worked especially hard to maximize the potential for her swallowing to return.

As spring moved into summer, we reluctantly accepted that her swallowing function would not be normal again. She had done her exercises with diligence through May, trying desperately to stimulate the nerves and muscles in her throat and neck so they would sync up and work properly.

But try as she might, her efforts didn't produce any meaningful results. And, as was the case with so many aspects of our life, accepting her fate was nearly as difficult as living with it. Acceptance had become a critical component of dealing with our lives. Doing so, we discovered, was essential to moving forward and functioning with some semblance of normal.

But doing so can chip away at your being. As Sara frequently said, she would never give up, but sometimes she had to give in. It was such a simple, yet poignant, perspective. And it accurately summed up so much of our lives.

While each of us knows the importance our culture places on mealtimes in a general way, it becomes painfully apparent when you are unable to eat. Sara often disappeared as dinnertime approached. I would look around and find she was nowhere to be seen, only to ultimately discover her sitting in our bedroom, watching television or reading.

As the weeks passed, she occasionally insisted that her swallowing function had recovered to a point that she was ready to try some food. After the first couple of bouts with this, I cringed when she said she would try it. I knew the outcome in advance. But I'd say nothing, realizing my protestations would just irritate her.

She would go to the refrigerator or cupboard and select some item, prepare it, and then sit down at the table—as we had for decades. After watching the pain of her first episode,

I chose to leave the kitchen, going to the family room so I would be close by, but not in her space as she attempted to eat.

She would fastidiously ready herself and then take her first bite. It was only a few seconds before she would begin coughing, often violently, as the residue from whatever she was eating slid toward her lungs, as well as her stomach.

It was no easy task, and her persistence amazed me. I could only imagine her mental anguish as she navigated her way through the detailed preparation. Eating was something she had successfully done thousands of times; now it sat atop the list of things she wished she could do. And, it was yet another loss.

When she was completely honest with herself, she understood the unfortunate truth that eating was no longer going to be a part of her life. Toss in the actual physical pain and frustration she experienced upon swallowing a bite, and it was amazing—yet heartbreaking—to watch.

Our life settled into a routine as I continued calling on clients, trying in vain to make my financial business work.

I was struggling with all aspects of it. Our income had shrunk to a fraction of what it had been. Sara was on Social Security disability. I had started my work in the financial world the previous August. While I had worked hard at it, my income was averaging somewhere around $3,000 per month. To put that in perspective, it was roughly twenty-five percent of what I had made per month while at CART. Making it that much more difficult, of course, was the fact we no longer had Sara's income.

Jenny was receiving a Social Security benefit, but because she was in psychiatric placement costing thousands a month, our arrangement with Easter Seals applied the entire amount of the benefit to her care.

I often had to resort to credit cards to pay for necessities. The pressure of it all was crushing and it greatly impacted our collective psyche. While my primary focus was on Sara and helping her fight the cancer, the pressures of being a caregiver; scrambling to pay bills' dealing with Jenny and her bipolar disorder; worrying about whether I would have a reoccurrence of cancer; and feeling disappointment about the work I was doing all combined to create a massive weight on my being.

Friends and some family members were supportive. I could sense they were awed by what I was enduring and it wasn't unusual to be asked how I was doing and told, "I don't know how you deal with all this. I couldn't do it."

My response was usually quick and genuine. "I don't really have much choice. I need to keep it together for Sara and our family. I'm not doing anything special. I bet you'd do the same."

No doubt, it wasn't easy. In fact, it was not only extremely stressful, it was a bit surreal. But I had one focus: to do the right thing for Sara and our family. She had always been there for us. I was determined to do everything I could to be there every day, every minute she needed me.

As summer ended, Sara was having more and more physical challenges. Each week, her balance deteriorated a bit more and it was obvious she needed assistance. Trying to anticipate the inevitable, I tracked down a walker and she sneered when I first brought it into our home.

"I'm not using that. I don't need it," she said dismissively as I showed it to her. "I get around fine. Get it out of here. Put it in the garage so I don't have to look at it. I don't want it in the house."

Less than a week later, she began using it to help get around.

I really understood, though. It was another concession, yet another subtle admission that the disease was winning. I shared her frustration and often wondered how I would behave if I were in her situation. Watching her slip away a little bit at a time became a sad, daily occurrence.

In early September, we visited Cancer Care for Sara's Herceptin and Zometa treatments. As we sat at the infusion center, she seemed particularly pensive and was very quiet. I mindlessly watched morning television and read a magazine as the treatment proceeded. The drug dripped into the port in her chest and, as her infusion was nearing completion, she voiced a rhetorical question.

"I'm really wondering if this is doing any good," she said, nodding toward the bag of liquid. "I don't think it's making any difference."

I looked at her and wondered where this was going, but knew she had a plan.

"My next appointment with Dr. Decker is next week," she continued. "I'll bring it up and see what he says."

The following Thursday, we met with her oncologist. He quizzed Sara as he examined her. She answered politely, but both of us knew she had more on her mind.

"David, I have a question for you," Sara said.

"You always seem to have a question for me," Dr. Decker replied with a smile, giving Sara a playful verbal jab. "What's on your mind?"

"Are these treatments doing anything to help me?" she asked.

Dr. Decker didn't seem surprised by Sara's question and went into his physician mode, as I expected he would. "Well, that's hard to say. Studies have shown Herceptin's benefits and—"

"David, tell me what you really think," she interrupted. "Let me put it this way: Would you stay on it if you were me?"

Dr. Decker paused for several seconds and then said, "Honestly, it's probably not making much of a difference."

Sara had the answer she was seeking. She embraced the moment and ran with it.

"You have always told me that, when I'm ready, you'll put me in hospice care," she said.

Dr. Decker was listening intently but said nothing as Sara continued.

"I'm ready."

In the space of the few seconds it took to have this friendly exchange, Sara had significantly changed the course of our lives.

She had decided it was time to give in.

"Of course," Dr. Decker said, offering no resistance to the idea. "I will make the arrangements."

We left his office with a surprising sense of newfound freedom. We had discussed this possibility before we went for the appointment, but could not have imagined how it would feel, once the choice was made. It was as if a weight had been lifted from us. The irony of the decision was not lost on us. We had admitted we were ready to go into the final steps of our adventure and we felt good about it. The struggle to get well was, at last, behind us.

But it was critical that Sara made the point.

"I'm not giving up," she said, almost defiantly. "But I *am* giving in.

"It's time."

That decision set a chain of events into motion. The day following our office visit, Beaumont's hospice organization contacted us and arranged for a representative to come by the house.

The next day, a hospice nurse came by and got the ball rolling. She started by taking Sara's vital signs and then discussed Sara's health status as she wrote in the chart. The nurse explained that another member of the hospice team would come by in a few days to drop off a bed and a few other items.

After she left, Sara and I looked at one another, considering what had just transpired and where we now were in our life together. The decision we had made was certainly a move toward closure on our long adventure. But more importantly, it provided us with relief—a lessening of the stress that we'd felt the past few years.

Sara looked me squarely in the eyes and offered the first comment. "I feel like a weight has been lifted off us. You can just feel it in the attitude of the nurse. There is no pressure. The battle to get well is behind me. I have to admit, I like that feeling."

It brought to mind all those who had, in their own way, tried to be supportive of Sara and our family over the years. The comments about "miracles" and "God's intervention" generally made me uneasy. But there were those who never backed away from that thinking. In a strange way, it reinforced the "giving up" thinking that created much of the unneeded external pressure and stress encountered when going through such an ordeal.

Hospice presented us with none of that. It was about getting and being comfortable. Accepting that death is a natural part of life. And getting there is not scary or some sort of dark secret that is meant to be feared. We both sensed that independence and it was a welcome addition to our lives.

We again felt we had some level of normalcy. We sat four times a day for Sara's feedings but, other than that, things felt more like they had several years earlier. Sara was able to get out and about a bit. The brain tumor had severely compromised her balance and stability but the walker was a crutch that allowed her to get around.

I took stock of our broader family situation, and it seemed to have reached a normal plane as well. Jenny remained at Havenwyck. It had been a year since she moved into the round-the-clock psychiatric setting. Sara and I had hopes that her first eighteen-month stint at Children's Home of Detroit would be enough, but Jenny's behavior remained erratic, at best. She had made some progress in her second placement, but it often felt like a one step forward, two steps back scenario.

Jenny's absence made it easier to manage Sara's illness and its accompanying issues. It also reduced the ongoing stress in my life. We both missed Jenny, but the endless confrontations and difficult situations we'd endured since the mid-90s had worn us down. We welcomed the relief that came with the separation.

Andrew had done well heading into his final year at Western Michigan. Sara and I were so proud of him. He was consistently on the Dean's List, had inserted himself into several aspects of the university's political science community, and had developed a serious, ongoing relationship. He made it home as often as possible, knowing that the time with his mom was running short.

My business was struggling, and the ensuing financial stress was relentless. It was something I hadn't considered as I had thought about caring for Sara. But it was a burden that played an ever-larger role, creating sleepless nights that, in turn, made it that much more difficult to focus on my responsibilities in caring for Sara.

My mom was around some and that was helpful. She had been slow to recover after my dad's death. I talked with her a couple of times a week, and she regularly told me how much she missed him. And while she loved being around us, she adamantly refused to drive the two hours from her home in Ohio to our place on the north side of Detroit because she disliked the heavy traffic. When she could, she would guilt one of my brothers into driving her to Troy to spend a few days. It was always great to have her with us.

With each passing week, Sara lost a bit more mobility, a bit more mental capacity and capability. The tumor in her brain was causing changes. Some were very noticeable, others small. But knowing her as I did, I noted even the slightest difference.

Her balance was getting worse by the day. She insisted on sleeping in our bedroom for the first couple of weeks after starting hospice care. But that hospital bed sitting in the soon-to-be-converted den/office downstairs was a constant reminder that it would become the place where she would spend her time.

The first week in October, we had a discussion about it.

"I really don't want to stop coming upstairs to sleep," she said. "I love our bedroom and bed. The bathroom is right here and, of course, it means I'm right next to you every night. But I'm afraid I might fall down the steps. I never really liked the steepness of them and they don't seem as wide, from front to back, as they used to. I never thought I would notice the narrowness of the staircase. It really helps to be able to lean against the wall when I'm coming down the steps."

Her unsteadiness on the stairs, and general shakiness, worried me. I agreed with her; I didn't want her to stop sleeping in our bedroom. It was yet another component of life slipping away. But the priority was keeping her safe and if that meant that she sleep downstairs, then that's what we would do.

Another concern was her taking a shower or bath. Since the lone bathroom on the main floor was a half bath, she had to go up the stairs to clean up. I'd made some changes to our second full bathroom, the one used by the kids. I added a handheld shower that allowed her to wash herself as she was seated on the shower chair I had purchased. I also had a couple of stainless steel bars added to help her remain steady as she maneuvered in the tub. It felt about as safe as we could make it.

During the first week of October, she made the decision to begin sleeping downstairs. It was not a stated decision. It just started. I breathed a sigh of relief that she no longer would be going up and down the stairs on a regular basis.

She insisted that I continue to sleep in our bedroom and I honored her request, even though I was uneasy about it. I worried about her falling when she got up during the night, went to the bathroom, or wandered around the house.

We had a discussion about her getting up during the night, and I told her I expected her to let me know (by using our cell phones) when she needed to get up. She said she would and did so for the first few nights following our conversation. I would rouse myself and get down the stairs as quickly as possible and help her to the bathroom. But that lasted only a few days before I was awakened to the sound of her walker banging against a wall as she tried to get it over the threshold from the hall to the bathroom.

I jumped from bed and raced down the stairs.

"What are you doing?" I asked, concern and a bit of annoyance in my voice. "We have an agreement that you won't come in here without me."

She mirrored my annoyance on her face before she spoke. "I'm *fine*. I can do this without you. You need your sleep and I know how tired you get. I'll be okay."

I was torn. I fully understood that she didn't want me monitoring her bathroom visits. It was yet another loss in her life. But I was terrified she would fall and bang her head on the corner of the counter or break an arm as she fell to the floor.

"I appreciate that you want to do this yourself, but our first priority is to keep you safe. I can't do that when you get up and come into the bathroom by yourself," I pleaded.

She clearly did not like my comments but bit her tongue and again agreed to call me before getting up from her bed.

The next day, as I ran some errands, I stopped at a store in search of an inflatable bed. I took the opportunity to lie on one and decided it was comfortable enough to work for me as a place to sleep downstairs. I made the purchase and took it home. As our bedtime approached, I pulled the large plastic bladder from the box, hooked up the electric pump, and watched as it grew to its fully inflated size.

"What's this?" asked Sara.

"I don't want you to fall and get hurt in the middle of the night. This way, I can sleep here on the living room floor, hear you get up, and help you."

She dismissed my concern, but I could tell she was happy we again would be near one another as we slept.

"I wish it would fit in the den so you could be right beside me," she said, a tired look coming over her face. "I really miss sleeping beside you."

"I know. So do I," I said. "But this will allow me to look up the hallway and into the den, so I can always be here for you."

She smiled and reached out to hug me. We embraced over her walker and she whispered to me.

"Down here or upstairs, you're always here for me. I know you are. It's such a wonderful feeling knowing that's so."

I put my arms around her and pulled her closer. I never wanted to let her go. She felt good in my arms and I felt good knowing she was confident that I would always be there for her.

She had lost so much. Making meals had given way to being fed through a stomach tube. Simple acts like getting toothpaste on her toothbrush and getting to and from the toilet required assistance. Reading had been replaced by watching television because she could no longer track along a page. She couldn't even get into her nightgown without help. And the rattle of the hospital bed safety rail being pulled up must have sounded like defeat every time she got into bed.

Sara's reduced energy level and deteriorating balance became a major concern as the weeks passed. I could no longer leave the house for work and feel comfortable.

I had to stay connected to my fledgling financial business, but I was struggling with being able to properly care for Sara. As I fought to grow my business, my boss thought it would be helpful for me to get out of the house, so at the urging of my superiors, I had taken office space a few months earlier. I understood his thinking, but I felt I'd been forced into it. I could spend a few hours there each day trying to get the struggling business off the ground, but it meant I had yet another expense at a time when I was juggling too many bills. When I was realistic with myself, I knew it would make little difference. My heart just wasn't into being a financial representative. My priority was to spend time with the wife I was slowly losing.

I had explored a few options regarding care for Sara when I was out. I spoke to the Beaumont hospice group about getting an individual to come to the house each weekday for four to six hours. But the cost was prohibitive under our financial circumstances, running upwards of thirty dollars per hour. I was discouraged but kept looking. Finally, I spoke with a member of the nursing staff who said she couldn't help me with any information but, with a wink, slipped me the phone number of a Detroit group that provided qualified personnel who were significantly less expensive.

I called and spoke to a woman who passed along the name and number of another person she recommended. I hung up, called the number, and talked with a woman named Toi who seemed very caring and nice. We set a time for her to come by the house the following day. I checked a couple of the references she provided, and when we met the next morning, I was quickly convinced she would be a good choice to help us. Following our conversation, she and I went in to talk with Sara. They hit it off from the start.

I felt a sense of relief as Toi arrived the next day and I left for my office. I tried, with some success, to focus on work and was able to spend more time on my clients. But I also checked in with Toi several times.

It went well. Sara really liked her.

I was relieved to hear Sara was pleased. Her care was my top priority and that would never change. But I worried constantly about my ability to juggle our cash flow and this had added another significant cost to the mix. It wore me further down, but I kept my concerns from Sara. We had always been upfront with one another about our finances, but I didn't want her to feel further guilt about her illness. In her down moments, she talked about how she was a burden. It was difficult to hear and I didn't want to do anything that would add to it.

Over the next few weeks, I watched as Sara's condition continued to deteriorate. She slept more, saving her energy for those occasions when she absolutely needed to get up. One of the few weekly obligations we kept was to meet with Jenny and her therapist at Havenwyck. We genuinely liked and respected the therapist and felt the sessions were helpful and moving Jenny in a positive direction.

One session in early November required us to get to Havenwyck through an unexpected snowstorm. Upon arriving, I parked in a handicapped space not far from the front door. The sidewalk was covered with a couple of inches of snow and huge snowflakes were falling at an ever-increasing rate. I was worried about Sara making her way into the building behind her walker. I got her situated outside the car amid the blizzard-like conditions and turned to lock the car. When I looked back, I saw her scurrying toward the front door, the wheels of her walker creating a wake in the snow on the sidewalk.

I was terrified she would fall on the concrete and raced up the walk, catching her as she reached the covered part of the path that led into the building.

"What are you doing, running off on your own in this snow?" I said, in a joking way but maintaining concern in my voice.

She pulled away from me and said, "I'm fine. I don't need you to help me every minute of every day."

It was the type of response that was not unexpected. I didn't challenge her but thought about how she could have ended up sprawled across the sidewalk, an arm or hip broken from the fall.

We went inside and she sat down in the waiting room, seemingly annoyed with my concern.

"I get worried about you, that's all," I said as I tried to maintain some calm, knowing she was annoyed with me. "It's snowing and you could easily have fallen. I don't want you to get hurt."

"I'm fine," she snorted with displeasure and turned to look out the window.

We waited a few minutes before going into Jenny's session. The hour went by quickly and we were soon headed back to the car. The snow had continued and the sidewalk was slushier than it was earlier. I took Sara's arm and held her as we slowly worked our way back to the car.

After we were situated inside and I started the engine, Sara turned to me and said, "Thank you for helping me into the car. I didn't want to fall and it could've happened if you hadn't held on to me. I'm sorry I got short with you."

I thanked her for the apology but said nothing more. I felt she had been demeaning to me and hoped she understood I didn't deserve to be treated with disrespect. It was a difficult juggling act. I had to balance Sara's illness and limitations with my need to feel appreciated and respected. I hoped she had gotten the message.

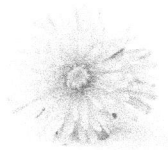

CHAPTER
16

Sara's personality and mood swings seemed to be increasing, sometimes making it difficult to spend prolonged periods of time with her. I knew the days we had together were numbered. Because of that, I wanted to spend every moment I could with her. But her rants about a variety of subjects—topics that just months ago would not have been on her radar—regularly made it difficult to be with her. It was such a departure for her and it was tearing me apart.

Early in November, she had told me how important it was for me to "be" with her. It wasn't a physical thing so much as one built on emotion. I wanted to honor her request and my concern in making it happen was a practical one. With her hospital bed and rolling tray, as well as a computer armoire, most of the space in the 11x12 room had been consumed. I wanted a chair that fit in the small space next to her bed but wasn't sure I could find one.

I searched for something that would work. It had to be lightweight, perhaps even collapsible. Most importantly, it had to be comfortable because I knew I would be spending countless hours in it. I found one I thought would work and bought it.

Sara was pleased to see I had been so quick to respond to her request. I pulled the chair from the box, set it up, and sat down. She smiled as I pulled the chair close, literally touching the side of her bed. It was more than a piece of furniture, it was a symbol of my commitment to staying close. And as symbols go, it was remarkably affordable—just fifty dollars.

Not everything in my life was as affordable as that chair, though, and some things came with more than a dollar cost. About a week later, I was sitting in the chair when I noticed that our dog Allie was acting strangely. As she walked down the hall toward me, she bumped up against the wall. She had always been an energetic, sometimes frenetic dog. I watched her closely and noticed she had begun to occasionally stumble. She seemed to be leaning to her left at times and the left side of her mouth was drooping slightly.

I tried to put it out of my mind but, over the next couple of days, the symptoms worsened.

I took her to our veterinarian and described her symptoms. He examined her, and then took an X-ray of her skull. The news was not good. She had a mass in her head that was pushing on her brain, giving her symptoms not unlike those associated with a stroke.

I was stunned. Would it ever end? Another tumor in our lives, creating havoc. The irony was crushing. Sure, Allie's a dog, but my mind quickly went to the kids. I was concerned about how this would impact them, especially with their mom so ill.

Surgery was possible, but it would be a delicate procedure costing several thousand dollars. I immediately thought about Andrew. Allie was his dog and losing her would be extremely difficult. I asked the vet if there was anything else we could do to help her.

"Well, as the mass grows, her symptoms will get worse," he said. "One thing we could do is give her some steroids. That should reduce the swelling and give her some short-term relief."

Andrew would be home for Thanksgiving break in about a week and the steroids sounded like a good option.

"How long would the effects of the drug last?" I asked.

"About a week," he said.

"I think I'll want to do that," I said, "as long as she isn't suffering. I'll bring her back before my son comes home for Thanksgiving break and get the shot."

I could tell he felt my pain.

"I'm sorry you are faced with this," he said. "I know your wife is very ill and adding Allie to that is tough, especially for your kids."

Allie was such a loving and fun dog. It was hard to watch her stumble around the house over the next week. Like Sara, some days were better than others for her but on the whole, her condition worsened.

I took her back a couple of days before Thanksgiving for the injection. The result was almost magical. Within the hour, Allie was nearly back to her old self. Her energy level soared and she was racing around like she always had.

I met Andrew the following day at the train station. I brought Allie with me and she lavished him with sloppy kisses. Over the Thanksgiving holiday, they had some good times together. We talked about the situation when I took him back to the train station that Sunday.

"I wish Allie could be this way indefinitely," I said, "but, as we discussed, when the steroid wears off, she'll be back to her true self, struggling. And it's only going to get worse. We don't want her to be suffering and I think we should plan to put her down."

He looked straight ahead and was quiet for the next several seconds.

"I know, Dad," he said. "She's been such a great dog. I hate to think we have to do this, but I understand." He paused for a few more seconds before continuing. "Can we wait until I'm home for Christmas break? I want to be here for her. Do you think she can do okay until then?"

His response was just as I expected: both caring and pragmatic. I promised to take care of her.

The next few days passed and, almost to the hour, her week of steroid influence ended and the left side of her mouth drooped, her energy level diminished, and she began to bump into things. We did all we could over the next couple of weeks to help and comfort her as her condition continued to decline.

I made an appointment with the vet for two days after Andrew returned from school and we approached the day with dread. Sara struggled to say good-bye, crying as we scooped up Allie to take her away.

Andrew placed her in the backseat of the car where they sat together as we drove the short distance to the vet's office. I had picked up Jenny and she came along, sitting in the front seat with me. At the veterinarian's office, we waited with anxiety, knowing we had but minutes left with Allie.

Once in a treatment room, the vet stepped aside as we said our good-byes. Tears flowed freely as we petted her beautiful, golden coat, telling her it was okay. We listened vacantly as the doctor told us how Allie would experience no pain, that it was like going to sleep. I wondered how many times he had done this and how difficult it was for him to see families struggle with their emotions as they put a pet down.

He turned away and picked up the syringe that would end Allie's life. Andrew had positioned himself directly in Allie's face, the two of them nose to nose. Tears were streaming down his cheeks. Jenny and I stood behind the table and the vet approached Allie, searched for a vein in her left front leg, swabbed the area with alcohol, and gave her the injection. Her eyes closed, a few seconds passed, and she twitched a couple times. Just that quickly, her life was over.

The vet slowly turned away, placed the syringe on the counter, and turned back to us to offer his sympathy. He told us to take as much time as we wanted and he left the room. Andrew sobbed quietly as he kept his hand wrapped around Allie's neck for a few more seconds and then he rose and moved away. Both Jenny and I were crying and stroked the yellow fur on Allie's motionless body. Suddenly, she twitched again as her muscles relaxed and Jenny was alarmed.

"Dad, is she really gone?" Jenny asked. "Is she dead?"

I tried to compose myself so I could answer. "Yes, she's gone. She could twitch a few more times as her body relaxes completely. It's okay, Jen. She's better off now. You saw how much she was struggling to get around. She had trouble keeping food in her mouth. She was crashing into things when she walked. She would fall. That's not the Allie we knew and not the one we want to remember. She would want us to think of her running, retrieving sticks, and playing. That is what we should always remember about her."

Jenny seemed fascinated in the moment and lingered over Allie for a while longer. One of Jenny's early diagnoses had been obsessive-compulsive disorder, and she seemed just a little too focused on Allie's body.

Andrew moved to her side, put his arm around her, and said, "Jen, come on. Let's go. It's okay."

We slowly turned and left. Amid the sound of quiet sobs, we made the short drive home and gathered around Sara in her small room. Her eyes, too, were red from crying, and we spent the next few minutes processing our feelings. Talking little; crying a lot.

Afterward, I thought of how the kids had handled the loss of their beloved pet. It was a touching, sad, and telling moment.

I wondered what the scene would be like in the coming days.

Christmas was quickly approaching and I had begun to make scaled down preparations for our holidays. Sara was always looking for ways to celebrate the positives in life, and soon after Andrew was born, she had begun to gather small items that were symbolic of various times of year. By the time we had moved to Michigan, she had several plastic bins full of those items. What she did with them was a constant reminder of why life is so grand.

Sara had bought an artificial Christmas tree and placed it in the foyer. Each month, she brought out a different grouping of "ornaments" to decorate the tree. January was skiing and winter sports. June, a time for summer items. December found the tree covered with miniature board games and Christmas ornaments. She was constantly on the prowl for such items and by the end of 2004, she had more themed groupings than months.

The tree had become one of the things many people mentioned when they spoke of Sara. It was a unique, creative, and memorable symbol that represented much of what she stood for.

Sara had always made Christmas a big deal in our home. We had a large, artificial, pre-lit tree, and it was always dripping with a couple hundred ornaments. I would have to manage Christmas this year and it felt a little overwhelming. Trying to juggle my work and be with Sara consumed almost all my time. I had little energy to devote to decorating for Christmas.

I talked with Sara and she understood. She told me we could just put up the tree and add a few ornaments. I was relieved she didn't expect me to do the outside decorations or the other stuff we annually placed around the house. She did say, though, that she wanted it to be a special Christmas, especially for the kids' sake. It went without saying that this would be her last holiday.

Over the next few days, I thought about how we could make it special. With all the Christmas paraphernalia we had, it was easy to get swept up in the "stuff." In my attempt to reach a "less is more" space, I landed on what I thought was a good solution. We'd go to church on Christmas Eve and return home to the barren tree. We would then make decorating the tree the focal point of our evening. Each of us would pick through the large container of ornaments and choose five to put on the tree. We would then place them on the tree, one at a time, explaining why each was chosen until we had placed our five ornaments.

The new process created several poignant moments as the ornaments were selected and hung. We laughed, cried, and hugged as the tree came to life. Compared to previous years, it looked a little sparse, but Sara put it all in perspective saying, "This is the best Christmas ever. It's just wonderful to be here. Each of us sharing our thoughts about the ornaments was very special."

Her comment did not ring hollow. We were fortunate she was with us for this one final Christmas.

Later in the week, we went to be with my family near Toledo. It was wonderful to see everyone and great to share some of our favorite comfort foods that only came out for the holidays.

Sara had very limited energy but insisted she did not want to miss the gathering. Watching the kids as they opened gifts was always a real treat.

As I took it all in, I noticed my mom sitting in the background, more quiet than usual. I sat down next to her and squeezed her knee. She looked at me and didn't speak right away. I could see a sadness in her eyes that I hadn't seen since my dad had died, more than two years earlier.

"I'm really feeling alone, more lonely than I ever have," she said, her eyes growing moist. "I don't know what it is, but I'm really feeling it."

She seemed genuinely depressed, and I wondered if anything else had been going on in her life. I tried to buoy her spirits as I offered, "You need to come and spend some time with us. Sara loves to have you there, and you can help me with some of the stuff I'm dealing with. It'd be great to have you. Let's do it after the first of the year, okay?"

The suggestion seemed to brighten her spirits a bit and she said, "That sounds nice. It's always so good to be with you and Sara. And I love little Murphy. I miss not having a dog, you know."

She had a shih tzu prior to Dad's death, but it had become aggressive and they ended up having to put it down.

"Then let's do it," I said. "Maybe Nancy and Jeff can bring you halfway, and we can meet at the Red Lobster in Monroe and have lunch."

I knew the Red Lobster thing would close the deal. Mom's love for that restaurant was well known in our family. We often laughed as we talked about how she would ask for a second basket of biscuits, which she then wrapped in a napkin and stuck in her purse to later enjoy at home.

We left my brother's place and returned to Troy to enjoy the final days of the holiday break. Jenny was around for much of it and appeared to have made some progress in dealing with her bipolar disorder. And it was always good to have Andrew at home. Like any twenty-something, he spent a large amount of time with his girlfriend, as well as his friends. Regardless, his presence was welcome. I made a real effort to ensure he and his mom had time alone together.

We spent New Year's Eve quietly at home. Sara wanted to try to watch the ball drop on Times Square, but neither of us made it to midnight. Jenny was back at Havenwyck and Andrew spent the evening with his girlfriend. I was up early on New Year's Day, enjoying a cup of coffee and reading the paper when the phone rang. I figured it was a friend or family wishing us a happy New Year. Unfortunately, I was wrong.

My brother Steve was on the line and his voice was quivering. "Ron, I have some bad news. Mom has died. Her neighbor found her in her car in the driveway of her apartment.

She was slumped over the steering wheel with the car still running."

I moved the handset from my ear and took a deep breath. Had I heard right? Mom was gone? I felt a rush that made me lightheaded. My thoughts immediately turned to the previous Sunday and the last conversation I had with her. A sense of sadness settled over me as I thought again about how lonely she seemed. I was really looking forward to having her come to the house, and we had already made tentative plans to get her to Troy.

As was often the case over the past few months, my little buddy, Murphy, sensed something was wrong. He stood on his hind legs, pawing at my leg, prompting me to pick him up. I grabbed him and held him close as I shed some tears, thinking about how Mom had said she loved the little dog.

I went into Sara's room, sat down in my black chair, and composed myself. She was asleep and I was hesitant to wake her, but knew I must. I touched her arm and she opened her eyes. She looked into my face and asked what was wrong.

"I just got a call from Steve," I said. "Mom died during the night."

Like me, she was stunned. Tears came to her eyes and rolled down her cheeks. We hugged and cried as the reality sank in. I held Sara tightly and felt a wave of loneliness come over me. I let the emotions roll through me for a time before my pragmatic side took over.

I needed to get everyone together to prepare for Mom's services. Also, I was thrust into the lead role as executor of her modest estate. But first, I needed to tell the kids. Andrew and I hugged and shed some tears when I told him. But I knew Jenny would be another case.

Jenny and my mother had long had a special relationship. They developed a strong bond when Jenny was a toddler and the relationship grew as Jenny aged. In fits of rage aimed at Sara and me, Jenny would often say that Grandma was the only person who understood and truly cared about her. It was a big part of Jenny's histrionics when she was in the throes of one of her episodes. Sara and I took it with a grain of salt, but it was difficult to hear.

With the connection Jenny had with her grandmother, I knew I had to tell her face-to-face. I called the staff at Haven-wyck to let them know and tell them I would be coming by. Jenny and I met in a private office and I told her the news. She was devastated, sobbing between comments about how much she loved her grandma and how wonderful she was.

We gathered up some of her things and I took her home. It was good for the four of us to be together as we processed the loss.

Later that day, I talked again with my siblings and discussed the arrangements. There would be a viewing at a local funeral home, and the service would be later in the week at my mom's church. She would be buried in the plot adjacent to my dad in the cemetery on the west side of the town where she had lived most of her life.

Later in the week, the kids, Sara, and I made the trip to Wauseon for the viewing and service. We stayed with Sara's mother and attended the funeral the next day. I had written Mom's eulogy and delivered it during the service, as I had for my dad when he died. Several people approached me after the service and said how much they enjoyed my words and added they could never have done it, that it would be too hard to remain composed. I responded by saying that it was an opportunity to celebrate mom's life and honor her by sharing some positive stories and my love for her, just as I had done for my father.

We returned to Troy later that evening. My mind was working overtime. The kids and Sara were sleeping, and I wondered about our future as I sped along the interstate. One thing had become clear to me: I wanted Sara and I to be as prepared as possible for her service. We had discussed it more than once but needed to nail down several of the specifics. I knew Sara was certain about what she wanted: a traditional church service with hymns and verses. I also knew who she wanted involved and what they would be doing. But we had never formalized it and I knew now that we had to do so.

I also realized I had to complete the arrangements for Sara's cremation. As far back as college, we had talked about whether we preferred to be cremated or embalmed. We agreed then that we wanted to be cremated, and we had never wavered. I had to purchase an urn, I thought, and figure out the details of the cremation. I had to nail down all the particulars of the service and was driven to do so, sooner rather than later.

Andrew headed back to school the next day and I took Jenny back to Havenwyck. Sara and I were again alone when I brought up the need to finalize her arrangements. I was happy she was willing to talk about it and we did so over the days that followed. I had taken some notes during previous discussions and dug those out so we had a foundation from which we built our plan.

Sara wanted a traditional Lutheran memorial service. That would include the entire liturgy, communion, Bible verses, and music. I knew it was extremely important to her. I listened and offered little as she ran through the specifics.

I had tracked down a funeral service bulletin from our church and we used it as a guide. The difference was that, since Sara would be cremated, there would be no casket in the sanctuary. Sara had previously expressed her desire for the service to be on a Saturday. Many on her wide-ranging and long list of friends would want to attend. Several would need to make travel arrangements. She wanted to make it as easy as possible on those who would be coming, and she also wanted to minimize the time people might have to take away from work.

We finalized our plans and, as I started to share them with people at our church, I was surprised to discover that cremation made some of our church friends a bit uneasy. The church had indicated it was moving ahead with a program that seemingly endorsed the practice.

A few months earlier, the church council had started to go in a direction to develop a columbarium (a structure housing several niches in which urns/ashes are stored) in a small chapel in the church complex. They had researched the project and were about to finalize it. It was far enough along that I was prepared to purchase one of the niches for both Sara's and my ashes. That's when, seemingly out of nowhere, a few people in the congregation voiced concern, saying the chapel was not the place to house "dead people's remains."

So much for the Christian "ashes to ashes, dust to dust" point of view.

Suffice it to say, the episode was handled poorly. I couldn't believe there were actually people at our church who were against something with a centuries-old history. The closed-minded attitude disturbed me so much that, in the end, I chose to not participate in the columbarium project.

I contacted the Cremation Society of Michigan and they sent a brochure about their services. I called them back to discuss the specifics and set the entire process in motion.

Despite the incident about cremation, I wanted to honor Sara's wishes about the service being held at the church. So many of her friends were people she had become close to at the church. I discussed Sara's wishes for her service with the pastor. He said it all sounded fine and that we would execute the specifics when the time came.

"Having gone through your dad passing away, and now your mom, it really hit me how important it is to be prepared," Sara said. "Plus, this is my show. I want it the way I want it to be."

"I'm so glad we talked about this," I said. "It puts my mind at ease to know what we'll do and that it is what you wanted. Having it finalized also means it will be easier at a time when things will otherwise be difficult. Thank you for doing this."

She didn't immediately respond but then said, "You know, there is so little I could control over the past few years. I always said I wouldn't let cancer run our lives, and I think we have done well with that. That said, as much as you try, the illness ends up taking far more control than you want. With this plan, it gives me the last word. I really like that."

What a reflection of Sara's independent spirit. It was funny—and appropriate—that in her death, she would have the last word.

CHAPTER
17

The crushing, gray winter of 2005 was in full swing. It made our situation even more difficult to deal with.

Things were getting no better at work. My heart just wasn't in it. Each day reinforced how little time remained with Sara and how I wanted to be at her side. I lost more of her with each passing day. I was never quite sure what I would encounter as I walked into the room where her hospital bed sat, but I knew one thing for certain: it would not be better than it was the previous day. And that wore heavily on my being.

Since Sara's liver and brain metastases, I had been pulled in many emotional directions: anger, disbelief, frustration, sadness, acceptance. I'd experienced, and honestly felt, that I had dealt with each of the emotions that go with losing a loved one. Still, I had issues that were unresolved.

My pent-up emotions were often manifested while driving. To call me an angry driver was a bit of an understatement. Being the good son I was, I had learned my angry driving behavior from my dad. That was, no doubt, some of it. But some of it, I realized, came from a feeling that it was a safe place to release some of the angst I felt about losing Sara, not to mention my feelings about dealing with a daughter who was struggling with mental illness and my undigested emotions about my own bout with cancer.

Sara and I had spoken about my anger, and I told her I didn't like the way it felt.

"You know what I am going to tell you, don't you?" she said in 2003 when we first discussed it. "You need to talk to someone professionally. Find a therapist you like and talk to him or her."

She was right. I needed an outlet for all that was going on in my life. I needed someone who could objectively review the situation and offer suggestions on how to better deal with all I faced. I sought out and found a psychologist I ended up seeing for nearly two years. We met every three weeks or so, and he offered insights that were valuable and useful as I wended my way through my journey.

My most memorable session came as we were digging into my anger. I had told him I understood why I was angry. I had some major things in my life that were bound to make me mad. I also told him that I knew I was dealing with my anger through my driving. I was often embarrassed at the way I had behaved—the yelling, swearing, and occasional flip off of another driver. It was especially disturbing when I behaved in that way with Sara and the kids as passengers.

My therapist smiled and said it was not unusual for someone to handle their anger in such a way. He continued by offering a hypothetical situation to help me better understand so I could begin to mitigate it.

"Okay, so let's assume you are headed out to run an errand. You're driving east on the 696 expressway and are on edge, waiting—almost looking—for someone who will 'do you wrong' as you drive. You're coming to the Mound Road on-ramp. Unknown to you, sitting on it is a guy who is there solely to head onto the freeway and cut you off."

He stopped and looked me in the eyes before adding, "Does that sound realistic?"

I didn't have to think long before responding with a little laugh, "No, of course not. You make me sound like I'm almost being paranoid."

He leaned in and seriously replied, "That's the point, Ron. Keep that in mind when you're driving. It isn't a personal thing. It's not a competition. The car is a conveyance. It allows you to get things done. It's not about being wronged. It's not a game. When people make it so, it can become deadly."

I mentally savored his comments. It was a simple, yet insightful, observation. I took it to heart and from that day forward, I have often thought of his example when behind the wheel. The bottom line was that he helped me immensely, and not just with my anger while driving. His observations were useful in many ways as I did what I could to manage the feelings I had about my life and, in particular, the feelings that came with the thought of losing Sara. Therapy was a critical element of me being able to function as I did throughout the ordeal. I often found I was in that state of numbness I had first experience decades ago. I had come to minimize the swings in my mood—no highs, even if and when there was something to get enthused or excited about, and no lows, when things were frustrating or we learned yet another negative fact. That sense of numbness became a necessity for me. Being in that state allowed me to keep my head down and do what was necessary before moving to the next task. It may not have been the best way to do it, but it was the way I did it. And it worked for me as I forged along, dealing with Sara's condition, Jenny, our finances, and all the rest.

Sara's condition continued to deteriorate as the next several weeks passed and by the middle of March, I knew we were getting close to the end.

I was in my office on Tuesday morning, March 22, doing prep for client cases when my cell phone rang. I looked at the screen and recognized the number as that of our lead hospice nurse, Kim.

"Hello, Ron," she said, a very serious tone in her voice. "I just examined Sara. I called to tell you she is transitioning to the final stage."

She said something else but I didn't hear it. Kim and I had discussed this eventuality. I knew I would receive the call telling me that Sara was close to dying. But the gravity of what I had just been told stopped me cold.

"If you can be here the rest of the week, I recommend you do it," she added as I tried to focus on her words. "Sara asked me if I would tell you that she really needs and wants you here."

I thanked her and hung up the phone. We were at the end.

I flashed back to the call I took in Toronto that started this nearly twenty-two years earlier. It had been a very long road. I wondered what reaching the final destination would be like.

I packed my briefcase, told a couple of business associates what was up, and stopped at the front desk to inform the receptionist. She said she would pray for us.

When I arrived home I reached for the door handle and stopped before coming in from the garage. Reality was sobering.

I had visualized this moment many times, but, now that it had arrived, it felt different. This wasn't imagining the future, this was the future slamming its way into my present. Our present. The present of which Sara had little left. I needed a moment before going in.

"Ron, is that you?" Sara asked as soon as I stepped through the door.

"Yep, it's me," I said, trying to sound as upbeat and positive as possible. I turned the corner and faced her as she sat upright in her hospital bed. She looked good. Toi had helped her put on some makeup and I noticed she didn't seem so pale.

"Are you all right?" I asked.

"Yes, I'm good. Really good," she said and then smiled.

I was surprised to see her in such a good mood, considering the news her nurse had delivered. It was obvious she wanted to talk more about it, and I sat down in the chair adjacent to her bed.

"You know, we've been going through all this for so long. And I'm so tired of being sick and tired. I'm really ready for this. I think you are, too. It won't be much longer and, honestly, I'm so ready to go. It's God's plan and I'm at peace with it."

There was a radiance about her. She truly was ready for the end. We had spoken about it several times—what it would be like and how we would handle it. The fear of the unknown was evolving into reality and it was not nearly as scary as when we first discussed it.

"I'll be here for you. I'm not going to be doing any more work," I said. "Tell me what you want, what you need, and I'll take care of it."

She smiled and didn't hesitate.

"You're a wonderful husband," she said. "You have gone way over and above what most men would do and I love you so much for that. We've had such a wonderful life. And we did it together. We've really been partners throughout and that is the way it should be."

I fought to hold back my tears. She was right. We were great partners and had made a terrific life for ourselves, despite the adversities we faced. I leaned in and embraced her. We held one another for what seemed like several minutes and, when we pulled back, we looked at one another through tear-stained eyes.

"Just sit here with me in your little black chair," she said with a smile, patting me on the knee. "Be here with me. That's all I want."

As we stared ahead, my right hand reached for her left and our fingers interlaced. The television was on, a soap opera playing in the background, the audio turned low. We both looked toward the television but didn't see what filled the screen.

I sat for a while as she dozed off. I got up and made some phone calls. I wanted our families to know where things stood. I spoke to my brothers and sister. I talked to my mother-in-law. I also called a few of our close friends to let them know. And of course, I called the kids.

Andrew said he would be home as soon as he could get away from school. I called Havenwyck to inform the staff. They called back soon after and put Jenny on the line.

"Hi, Dad," she said with some hesitation, sensing this was different than most of our conversations. "The staff said you wanted to talk to me. Is everything okay?"

I took a breath and said, "You know how we've talked about Mom and when it's getting close to the end? The nurse says we're there, that mom is in the final few days."

Jenny was uncharacteristically quiet. After a few moments, she spoke as she began to cry. "She isn't going to die today, is she?"

"No Jen, it isn't that close. But I'll be getting you this evening so you can be here. We'll all be together."

I knew her next question and answered before she asked it.

"Andrew's coming home, too. We'll all be together for the next several days."

My phone rang frequently the next couple of days. Often, it was Sara's close friends—Beth, Terri, Suzie, Jules. They talked to Sara when she was able. The five of them had gone off annually the past few years for long weekends. They'd had the best of times. They had grown up together and always been close. As adults, each had gone her own way, but they had come back together in recent times to reconnect and enjoy the collective energy and fun they experienced together. It was always a time Sara relished, and she had again grown closer to each of them as time passed and her disease progressed.

They had last visited Sara in early September of 2004. They came together at our home, knowing it was probably the final time the group would include Sara. It was wonderful that they made the effort to come to Troy and clearly demonstrated the love they shared for one another.

I thought back to that time and how much I enjoyed seeing them. It was Saturday of Labor Day weekend and, as they were getting up, having coffee, and making breakfast I had to leave to take Andrew to his girlfriend's home in

Clarkston, about a half hour away. They were heading back to Kalamazoo for their fall term of college.

It was a gray and drizzly morning and traffic was heavy, heading "up North" for the final weekend of Michigan summer. I dropped off Andrew and headed south on I-75. As I came to the north edge of Great Lakes Crossing mall, out of the corner of my eye I saw a car slide sideways in the northbound lanes and bounce into the median. Mud and water flew as the car shot out of the grass and into southbound traffic. I hit my brakes and watched the incident unfold in slow motion before me. The car flew out of the median, landed on the pavement, and continued across traffic. As it got to the far right lane, a black SUV t-boned the car, pushing it back into the middle of the freeway. The sound was something I will never forget and pieces of metal, glass, and plastic rained down everywhere.

I came to a stop about fifty yards from the wreck. I heard screams from a woman who had been riding in the SUV. I pulled out my cell phone and pushed 911. An operator quickly answered. I gave her information as I walked toward the smoldering car. A small fire was burning in the rear. I hesitated but also knew that if the fire spread and there was a chance to pull someone out, I wanted to do so. My racing experience told me it was a small oil fire, so I continued towards the car. When I got to it and looked inside at the driver, I saw that it was a young woman, probably in her early twenties. The driver's side door and side post were crushed into her lifeless body. Her beautiful blue eyes remained open and had a hollow look of terror in them.

Life is so fragile, I thought as my eyes began to tear up.

But I was still on the line with the dispatcher.

"Sir? Are you still there?"

I broke my gaze on the crushed driver and tried to compose myself as I turned to walk from the car.

"Yes, I'm here," I said, sniffing as I tried to stifle my crying.

"You are the second person to call on this," the voice on the phone said. "We have dispatched emergency vehicles and they should be there shortly. Thank you for calling us."

"Okay," I said. "Unfortunately, I don't think there is much that they will be able to do for the driver of the car that was hit."

As my call ended, a man came running up to me. He told me he was an off-duty Detroit police officer and asked me if I was okay. I told him *I* was but the woman in the car looked like she hadn't made it. He continued toward the crushed car. I walked back to my vehicle, got in, and drove on the left shoulder around the carnage. The feeling of numbness I had felt so often had leapt back into my life. Sirens wailed from ambulances, police cars, and fire equipment as they passed me headed northbound to get to the surreal scene.

I returned to the house and told Sara and our friends of the accident. I had seen death swoop in and claim individuals at the racetrack, but this was different. An innocent young woman's life was snuffed out before my eyes.

That event flashed into my mind as I talked to Beth when she called to talk about Sara's final days. It made me think how tough Sara had been for more than twenty years through all of this. Her years of resilience had been extraordinary. But it also reinforced and vividly reminded me how, in a moment, a life can end.

The kids and I hunkered down and spent much of our time gathered around Sara in her small hospital bed during the next several days. Each time I sat down with Sara for her tube feeding was a special moment. As we had done hundreds of times, we sat knee to knee. It had become our intimate time. We savored those few minutes.

Sara's body was slowly shutting down and she slept most of the time. She moved from her bed only for feedings and to go the bathroom. Each of us took our turn helping her get up. It was difficult to see her in such a compromised state. Fortunately, she didn't seem to be in any significant pain. It was more a question of her energy level. She was just slipping away.

Sara's youngest sister, Cyndi, and her husband visited Friday. Sara was surprisingly lucid and even a bit feisty. I moved her into the special chair I had purchased for her a few months before. It was a club chair that was on the smaller side, and she said it was perfect because it fully surrounded—really enveloped—her. She said it made her feel warm and cozy.

As we talked with my in-laws, Sara chided me for "taking over and making all the decisions." We laughed about that and other memories from our collective past. After about forty-five minutes, I could sense Sara was wearing down and, being as protective as I was with her well-being, I suggested we move her back to her bed. She hesitated but knew it was where she needed to be.

After they left, Sara immediately fell asleep. I was hesitant to rouse her for feeding a couple of hours later. I understood it really made little difference in her condition. But I also knew we had so little time together and, selfishly, I didn't want to surrender that closeness and our brief intimate time together. I quietly got her up and brought her to the kitchen. It was good to be together, but she kept falling asleep as I held the syringe and tube to allow the liquid to slip into her stomach. I finished, got her back together, and moved her to bed. She was asleep as I finished covering her.

I sat at her side and watched a bit of television, and then brought out my inflatable bed. The kids were around but were tired, too, and we all went to bed as Friday wound down.

Our hospice nurse arrived around 8 o'clock Saturday morning, examined Sara and came to the kitchen to ask me how things were going.

"We're doing okay," I said. "It's been great to have all this time together. Your advice was right on and I'm so glad we have spent the week together. We've had some really wonderful quality time."

I was curious about what lay ahead.

"She doesn't have a lot longer," she said. "Just keep her comfortable and call us if there are any significant changes. We're there for you any time, day or night. Don't hesitate to call if you need something or just want to talk."

I walked her to the door and returned to Sara. I fell into the black chair and reached for her hand. It felt cold and clammy. I turned to look into her face. Her eyes seemed sunken into her skull, dark circles underscored her sockets, and her skin tone was slightly ashen. Her pretty brown eyes opened but didn't have the sparkle I had known for the better part of forty years.

"How are you doing?" I asked.

"Ready to not have to answer that question anymore," she said, her sense of humor shining through.

I laughed and squeezed her hand.

"Can I get you anything?"

"No," she said. "I'm okay." She was silent for a couple of minutes before she again spoke. "Do you have any regrets? Has our life been all you wanted?"

I answered without hesitation. "Our life has been terrific. We have had such a great run. As we always say, we have had so many great adventures, wonderful times together, and I wouldn't trade any of it." I stopped but then added, "There is one thing I would have changed."

Sara looked at me, confusion registering on her face. "Really? What's that?"

"I wish we weren't where we are today," I said. "I always looked forward to growing old with you, seeing the kids off on their lives—together. I don't relish having to do it alone. I wish we would have been able to do it together."

She squeezed my hand. Weakly, but a loving squeeze, nonetheless.

"I know," she said. "I would like to be here for that, too. But I know you'll be everything to the kids that we would have been together. I'm comfortable with that."

We fell silent for a few moments before she asked another question.

"Are you okay with Jenny coming home and being here full-time?"

"I think she has made good progress," I said. "I believe she is ready to be here. Honestly though, I don't know how I could've taken care of you as I have and had Jen here. It would have been difficult. It's weird how things work out, and the timing of this has been good."

We had talked for the past couple of months about Jenny being discharged. The target date was mid-April. Sara had managed to hold on for a few more months than most in her situation would have. I had often thought that was so she could see Jenny back at home. She wanted to leave comfortable in the fact Jenny would be okay.

My mother-in-law and Sara's oldest sister arrived that afternoon. I brought Sara from her bed to her club chair in the family room. Her energy was nearly gone, compromised to the point that she had trouble holding her head up. She spent most of their visit sleeping.

I carried the conversation. Sara offered no more than four or five sentences during their visit. My sister-in-law, Ann, rose after about an hour and said they probably should go. They each hugged Sara, who was barely able to rouse herself to say good-bye, and I walked them to the door. Then I helped Sara back to her bed. I almost had to carry her into the room just a few steps away. I got her into bed and she was asleep as her head hit the pillow.

Our hospice nurse checked in, asking if there had been any changes. I told her Sara's energy level was evaporating at an increasing rate, that she had trouble just lifting her head. She said that this was not unusual and that I should concentrate on making certain she was comfortable.

Like me, the kids were worn down from the past few days. Jenny stayed at Sara's side almost nonstop and Andrew, looking for a few moments to clear his head, decided to go out with a couple of his friends. I put my inflatable bed into position so I could peer down the hallway as I had for the past couple of months. I was exhausted. The week had completely worn me down and most of it was mental. I crawled onto the bed and immediately fell asleep.

Around 2:00 a.m., Andrew shook me awake. He sounded a bit panicky, saying his mom's breathing was loud and strange. I heard the raspy sound in the distance. It sounded like Sara was gasping with every breath and we hurried to her side. We shook her awake and she sleepily opened her eyes but didn't speak.

Andrew and I were getting frantic, wondering what to do to ease her ragged breathing. I remained as calm as I could but it was difficult to do. I decided to call hospice. I described the situation and the woman on the other end spoke in a very measured way, which was very reassuring.

"Ron?" she said, "just slow down a little. It will be okay. You have the kit we gave you when Sara started hospice, right? It's in your refrigerator, I assume?"

I answered that it was. She directed me to get it and I walked to the refrigerator, opened the door and found the small cardboard box I had positioned on the top shelf in a back corner. I brought it back to the counter near the phone.

"Inside the kit is a small bottle with a liquid that should help her. Do you see that?" she asked.

"Yes, I have it here," I said.

"Good. What I want you to do is take it to Sara and put a couple of drops under her tongue. That should allow her to breath more normally," she said. "It will help pretty quickly."

Andrew and I took the small brown bottle and grabbed a phone handset from another room so I could continue the conversation. We worked together to open her mouth and dripped a couple drops under her tongue.

"Okay, we've done it," I said to the woman on the phone.

"Do you notice any difference?" she asked.

Sara's breathing seemed to almost immediately become less labored. She appeared to relax and breath more deeply and less often.

"Yes," I said. "It seems to have helped her."

"Good. Now, take the oxygen machine, put the nosepiece into her nostrils and turn on the machine so oxygen is flowing. That will help, too. Continue to monitor her breathing and when it becomes difficult again, give her some more drops from the bottle," she added. "One of our nurses will be out to see you around 8:00 or so this morning."

Andrew and I were relieved we'd been able to provide Sara with some comfort.

"Do you have any other questions?" she asked. "Do you feel you're doing okay?"

"No more questions. I think we're fine now," I said, relieved. "I was so worried. She was struggling and I wondered if we would be able to help her."

"That's normal," she said. "Don't worry about it. I'm glad you called and that I could help. Don't hesitate to call again if you have any other questions."

I hung up the phone, went back to Sara's bedside, and plopped down in my chair. Andrew was sitting on the edge of Sara's bed. I reached over to hold her hand. It seemed cold and I put my hands around it to warm it up. I turned on the television to mask the humming sound of the machine pumping oxygen to Sara's face. Andrew looked as tired as I felt, and I told him to go to bed, adding that I would come get him if anything changed. He bent down to hug Sara, he and I hugged, and then he reluctantly went to bed.

My fatigue overwhelmed me and I soon fell asleep and awoke at dawn's light. Sara had not moved since we had placed the drops on her tongue. Her breathing was less labored than it had been but was again getting ragged. I placed a couple more drops under her tongue. I struggled to wake up. I felt I was both watching a film and was one of the actors in it. After all we had experienced the past couple of days, it was too early to wake the kids, but I knew they would want to be with their mom. The developments overnight made me wonder how to handle the situation with them. I didn't want them to feel left out of the vigil. And the last thing I wanted was for them to miss being with their mom during her last moments. I knew I would always regret it if Sara died while they were sleeping.

As I thought about that, my mind considered the actual moment when someone dies. I flashed back to the day my father passed away in 2002. He went fairly quickly after being diagnosed with metastatic lung cancer. All his years of smoking had caught up with him. My mom had made few plans to prepare for losing him, and we, my siblings and I, spent much of his last couple of days making calls, preparing paperwork, and thinking about what else needed to be done.

My brothers and sister, our kids, and my mom had filled their small, two-bedroom apartment, maintaining a vigil as my dad lay dying in a hospice bed in their small dining/living room. While everyone else surrounded my dad, I was in their spare bedroom. Someone had to write his obituary and get it off to the funeral home and the local newspapers. That task fell to me as the writer in the family. I wondered how many family events I had missed throughout my life as I traveled the world, banging out stories on my computer, doing what needed to be done during my career in sports.

I finished the copy and was reviewing and editing it when one of my sisters-in-law opened the door and told me dad was gone. In the years that had passed, I occasionally wondered if I should have been at his bedside when he drew his last breath.

The hospice nurse arrived on schedule, took Sara's vital signs, asked a few questions, and quietly told me that she didn't think Sara would make it through the day.

She asked me if I had any questions. I told her no but that the kids and I had wondered if Sara could hear us when we talked to her.

"It's hard to say," she said. "There is research that suggests patients in their final few hours can hear those speaking to them, even if they appear to be asleep, or even comatose. I'd say you should talk to her, figuring she can hear you."

I told her thanks and I walked her to the door. She turned to me as she was about to step outside. "She seems comfortable," she said. "Don't hesitate to use some more drops if she starts to struggle. Comfort is the number one priority now. And as we always say, you can call us if you have any questions."

About that time, Andrew came down the stairs and wondered how Sara was doing. The nurse recounted what she had told me.

Andrew and I returned to the small room, and I stood so he could sit in the bedside chair. He pulled up close to the bed and turned his attention to his mom, holding her hand. I left him with her and his thoughts.

As the day moved along. Andrew's girlfriend joined us, as did Sara's friend, Marilyn, and her husband. Our pastor came by, too, and spent a couple of hours with us after saying a few prayers over Sara. We anticipated that Sara could go at any time.

The last rays of sunlight slipped away and Sara's condition remained the same. She had only once started gasping and I used the drops from the brown bottle to again quiet her breathing. The evening turned to night and Sara continued to soldier along.

We went through the night with little sleep, spending most of our time at Sara's bedside. We talked about how appropriate it was for Sara to hang on as she was. It was so much like her to beat the odds laid out by the medical folks and, again, she was doing so. Night turned to day and the hospice nurse again appeared and examined Sara. She mentioned how surprised she was that Sara had made it this long but added she didn't expect her to linger much longer.

That morning, Sara gasped a couple times and it startled us. I gave her more drops and it seemed to help. We sensed that we were closing in on the last few hours. The funeral home called just before 10:00 a.m. I stepped out of the room to talk to them, leaving the kids with their mom. We had been gathered around her, providing comfort and saying it was okay for her to go.

I was looking at the huge oak tree in our backyard, the phone pressed to my ear, when I felt a hand on my shoulder. Toi, who had called me early that morning wondering about Sara, had come to the house. She wanted to be with us in Sara's final hours.

Her tap on my shoulder startled me and I turned to see her crying.

"She's gone," she said quietly, tears running from her eyes.

I told the woman on the phone I had to go and hung up. I started to cry as Toi and I hugged and then I went in to see

Sara lying there, her eyes closed, chest no longer rising to capture a breath. Andrew had left the room but returned with Laura. We gathered around Sara and hugged her and one another as we cried.

"I was the only one with Mom when she died," Jenny said as tears rolled down her cheeks. "I'm so glad I was with her at the end."

It was special for Jenny to have been the only one to be with Sara when she died. I told her that her mom would have liked it that way. It seemed to be a point of comfort for her. We spent the next few minutes at Sara's bedside, consoling one another and agreeing that it was best she was gone.

Death is a strange phenomenon. It comes in so many ways: quickly, quietly, violently, peacefully. I thought about how it had come to Sara. While she had moments of struggle and her breathing, at times, was labored and difficult to watch, in the end, Sara's death came peacefully. Her body just stopped. There was no drama, just her moving to the next chapter.

I called the funeral home, and when I reached the woman I had spoken with earlier, she said she would dispatch their people to the house to pick up Sara's body and take it to their facility. About a half hour later, two men in their thirties came to the door and said they were there from the funeral home. I showed them in and they surveyed the room before retreating to the white Chrysler minivan they had backed into the driveway. They returned with a heavyweight cardboard, coffin-sized box. The kids and I sat in the family room as they placed Sara's body in the box. They walked down the hall carrying her in the box and took Sara past her tree in the foyer one final time before they left the house through the front door. I watched from the garage as they loaded her body into the minivan, closed the tailgate, and slowly drove away.

As the van slipped out of sight, it struck me how anticlimactic the past hour had been. A wonderful and full life had ended fifty-two years and five months, to the day, after it had started.

Sara never gave up.

But she had finally given in.

CHAPTER
18

The three of us were exhausted. We spent much of the remainder of the day consoling one another and we went to bed early.

We began to plan for Sara's memorial service the next day. I had the outline Sara and I had created and it served as the framework to follow. I had talked with our pastor when he was at the house two days earlier about doing the upcoming service, which we would do Saturday.

As Andrew, Jenny, and I talked, we thought about how we could make the service the very best to honor the memory of their mom. I had collected several photos I wanted to use in a video tribute to start the service. I chose two pieces of music. Sara loved Doris Day's rendition of "Que Sera, Sera," and it was to play during the first couple of minutes of images. The Beatles' "The Long and Winding Road" covered the rest of the photos.

We also wanted to create a memory card that people would take away from the service. I pulled together the copy, and Jenny, who had taken a class in calligraphy with her Grandma Richards, used her skills to dress up the card. It ended up being a unique and nice personal tribute to Sara.

I spoke to Sara's siblings and mother about the service and the roles they would play. As I had with my mom and dad, I chose to deliver Sara's eulogy. I knew it would be difficult, but I did not want it any other way.

We talked about how we could further personalize the service and, as we did, we decided that Sara's celebration tree must be part of the tribute. I talked with our pastor about the idea and he agreed it was such a symbol of Sara's approach to life that it should be front and center in the church sanctuary.

I told the kids of this development and our next chore was to decide which decorations to place on the tree. We pulled several of the plastic bins from the front hall closet and went through the ornaments, reminiscing often as we poked through them. We ended up choosing those Sara had regularly used to announce the start of spring.

Later that day, Jenny came to me and wanted to talk.

"Dad, I've been wondering about the tree and the ornaments," she said.

"What're you thinking?" I asked.

"I'd like to put words on the tree that tell people about the kind of person Mom was."

"Wow, Jen" I gushed, "I think that's a great idea! How do you want to do it? How will you create the words?"

"I thought I could do it on the computer."

I hugged Jenny and told her how much I thought Mom would like that. She smiled and said she thought she would, too.

The three of us remained very busy as we prepared for the service. It was good to be able to do something that took our thoughts away from our loss. I spent a large amount of time on the phone. Sara's lengthy list of friends sprang to life in her passing, everyone wanting to talk about her dying and how much they admired her determination and fight. It was comforting to hear from so many people. Most conversations included both moments of laughter and a few tears as we caught up. Most said they would try to get to Saturday's service. As I considered the positive responses from those who said they would be there, I began to wonder if the church would be able to accommodate everyone.

There was one thing that was making me a bit anxious. Sara's cremation was scheduled for Wednesday afternoon, and I had arranged for the kids and I to visit the crematorium. It was out of the ordinary for a family to go to the cremation site, but I felt it would help Jenny process Sara's death by getting answers to the questions I suspected she would pose. We met one of our church's assistant pastors and headed to the western suburbs of Detroit. We were quiet as I drove to the location, a nondescript area populated by a seemingly endless number of small businesses specializing in light industrial work.

I drove through a long line of concrete, prefabricated buildings and came to the address we were seeking. We were greeted by a pleasant man in his mid-thirties who had several piercings and was covered with tattoos. He smiled and invited us into his garage-like area. My eyes immediately went to the large cardboard box that sat partially exposed in a large metal object.

"Please, come in," he said. "I'm very sorry for your loss. Sara is over here."

We walked the short distance to the container. A twelve-inch square of the box had been cut away, and as we looked in, we could see Sara's face. She looked like she was sleeping, no different than when she died. She wore the nightgown she had on when they had taken her away.

We gathered around the foot of the box and the pastor led us through the next few minutes. We joined hands around the makeshift coffin and he said a prayer to start the casual service. He read a couple of Bible verses before closing with another prayer, then stepped back to give the kids and me space to say our final good-byes.

Andrew and I had roses and Jenny had Sara's favorite flowers, daisies. We place them in the container. The kids had also written notes. They placed them under Sara's chin alongside the flowers. We stood over her for a few more moments, getting our final look at the woman who had meant so much to the three of us. I had an arm around each of the kids as we said a final good-bye, and then I steered us away from the container.

Primarily for Jenny's sake, I asked the crematorium operator to describe the process. He didn't hesitate to explain that the industrial furnace reached a temperature that approached 1800 degrees and that the cremation would take somewhere between 1½-2 hours. Sara's ashes would be collected and placed in a heavy plastic bag that would be closed with a metal tag that ensured the right ashes were given to the proper family.

As we left, I wondered how many families he had educated about the process. His thorough approach was sensitive yet impressive. We thanked him for the explanation and slowly left. We all seemed to be wrestling with our thoughts as we drove home. An occasional bout of quiet crying was the only sound that broke the hum of the car on the freeway.

Later that evening, the kids asked why their mom and I had chosen cremation. I told them we'd made the decision when we were in college. In the idealistic days of the early '70s, we agreed that it was selfish to take up ground in a world that would someday be pressed for space. Cemeteries, we thought, were space that could be put to better use. Also, Sara always had a thing about being cold and, for some reason, she had decided that her body not being in the ground would remedy that.

I also explained that Sara and I had discussed six places where she wanted some of her ashes spread. Round/Devils Lakes in Michigan, where we had spent a week every summer since moving to the Detroit area, was one of those places. The farm in Wauseon, where Sara grew up, was another. Our backyard in Troy, the Colorado State campus where Sara and I went to college, the foothills overlooking CSU on the banks of Horsetooth Reservoir near Fort Collins, Colorado, and the park in Thiensville, Wisconsin, across the street from the first place we lived in the Badger state—these spots were all special to her. I'd assured her that I would see to it that her ashes were spread at each spot.

Beth, from Sara's close circle of friends, called on Tuesday to offer her condolences. We had visited she and her husband in downtown Chicago on our "Lap of Lake Michigan" trip. She informed me they had long ago planned a trip for the upcoming weekend and would not be able to make Saturday's memorial service. Beth felt terrible and told me she wanted to come to Troy Thursday to spend time with the kids and me. I told her that while we had a few loose ends we would be securing, it would be wonderful to have her.

She arrived Thursday morning and we spent several hours reminiscing. It was time I cherished and it gave us a break from the singular focus we had on the details of the service.

Saturday morning came and we were up early for the service. The kids and I got into our Sunday best and headed to the church for the mid-morning service. I expected a big turnout. It ended up being even larger than I anticipated. As we neared the 10:00 a.m. start, I peeked into the sanctuary and was surprised to see ushers placing folding chairs at the back of the church. That meant there were around three hundred people in attendance. I smiled to myself, knowing Sara would have been humbled but happy by the turnout.

When it came time for me to deliver the eulogy, I walked to the podium and spoke for about five minutes on something we all knew—how special a person Sara had been—but needed to hear again. And again. It was all part of the grieving process each of us was experiencing. I finished without breaking down, although I had tears in my eyes as I walked back to my seat in the first pew.

After the service, many people recounted how profoundly Sara and her "never say die" attitude had impacted them and how inspiring they had found her. It was a source of great comfort to realize how many people's lives she had touched.

The program was not entirely complete, though. A Lutheran service usually concludes with a meal that is served in the church's community area, and this was no exception. During that time, dozens of people came to me to share stories, offer their sympathy, and give the kids and me hugs. As it was winding down, I could feel exhaustion consuming me. But it was one of those good exhausted feelings—like that glow Sara and I had many times felt after a long day of skiing.

My siblings, as well as Sara's family, retired to our house. Somehow, more food appeared and we shared many more memories and moments, recalling great stories from the past while occasionally breaking down. In the end, I was very torn. I was so tired I could barely stand up. I both wanted and didn't want people to leave.

As the sun set, it was only the kids and I at home. My mind was overflowing with wonderful memories from the day. That was no surprise; Sara engendered those kinds of thoughts.

Among those memories, though, was how uncomfortable people seemed in offering condolences. Many times during the day, I felt as if I was the one comforting them.

Sara would have liked that.

It hit me, too, how different life was going to be. In a couple of weeks, Jenny would be discharged and at home with me. I also knew I had to make a change in my career path. All that would come, but in due time.

The kids and I were really ready to catch up on our sleep. On Sunday, Andrew would be going back to school and Jenny would return to Havenwyck. After the kids went to bed, I picked up around the house. I finished and sat down in the family room. I looked around and realized that Murphy was upstairs with Jenny. I was alone—very alone. I sat for a few moments and absorbed the feeling. A sense of incredible emptiness settled in, kind of like a sheet that someone shook out and then let slowly fall down over me.

I had a huge feeling of relief knowing that Sara was no longer struggling. But it really hit home that she was gone.

And then I started to cry. It started slowly but quickly changed to a hard, from the diaphragm, kind of cry. When I finally composed myself, I was completely spent. It felt good and I trudged up the stairs to go to bed.

I thought about my loneliness again as I brushed my teeth. It had been five days since Sara died, but something was different that night. It seemed so final. I had been so busy, so occupied, preparing for the memorial service, and now that it had passed, I realized that the next stage of life was truly beginning.

Sara had often said that I would move on, find someone else, and settle down. It was too soon for that, but I did wonder where life would lead. It was certain, I thought, that it would be an adventure. This time, though, it would be without the woman I had loved for nearly forty years.

The next few days passed and loneliness consumed me. It felt empty—and so lonely. I had done virtually nothing since the service. Certainly, I'd done nothing that seemed productive. A massive hole had appeared in my life. The turmoil and activity that comprised the days following Sara's death had been such a welcome diversion. Planning and executing our memorial service plans, talking with friends and family, and the service itself had kept me focused.

Now it was time to begin another new normal. Andrew would soon be off to live and work in Washington, DC. Jenny was set to transition from Havenwyck to live at home again. It would all be very different.

Even though Sara had been largely "absent" during the last few months she was alive, her presence was an important component of my day-to-day existence. She often wasn't very lucid. And she often didn't feel like interacting. Her absence was far more impactful than I ever expected. The house had Sara's fingerprints all over it and that was even more vivid to me as I sat in the family room with our little shih tzu.

As I evaluated where I was, I accepted that I was exhausted. The events of the past five years had been far more draining than I'd ever admitted to myself or even realized. I had known it on some level, but now I was coming to intimately understand it.

Being the primary caregiver for someone who is dying is incredibly stressful—a reality often lost in the scheme of things as it all unfolds and a life is ending. I had little time to catch my breath during those five years, and I was now grappling to fill gaping holes in my days. I felt little motivation and accepted that I was depressed. I had trouble sleeping, no appetite, and little interest in doing much of anything. I made an appointment to see Dr. Khilanani, who prescribed an antidepressant for me. It took a while for it to work, but when it did kick in, I didn't like the foggy and sluggish feeling it created and stopped taking it.

And then there was my future. I had many moments of wondering where I would go from here and what life would hold as I went forward. I had many questions, but no answers.

When Sara entered hospice, I discovered that grief counseling was offered for several months following the death of a loved one. I had a good amount of experience with therapy and had always embraced it. I had used counseling to overcome issues more than once in life and I knew that it would now be a big help.

I dug through the hospice paperwork, found the phone listings, and contacted the Beaumont hospice therapy center to make an appointment. My counselor was a social worker, Ann, who I liked immediately. I began unloading my story in our first few hour-long sessions.

As the second meeting was ending and I was concluding my account of what had gone on, a long silence filled the room. Ann scribbled a few final notes and then stopped and stared at her note pad for several seconds before she spoke.

"Whew, Ron," she said, "you have endured so much the last several years. Frankly, it's amazing to me that you've done as well as you have. I'd say you've emerged in relatively good shape."

I looked down at the floor for a few moments and then up at her. "That's easy for you to say," I said, trying to make a joke before quickly getting serious. "I've done okay with all this, but I certainly don't feel anything near what I would consider normal. I vaguely remember normal, but I'm not sure I would recognize it."

She paused again, surveying her notes before she smiled and said, "That's because normal has evolved. You have a very new normal. The sooner you get your head around that and accept it, the sooner you will be able to move forward."

As time passed, Ann and I discussed much about how I had—and hadn't—grieved Sara's death. Over the ensuing weeks, I made decent progress. Then she offered a very poignant observation.

"I've listened to you for a few weeks now, heard about all you did, about how you tried to manage it all. And I have to say, for the most part, you did a fantastic job."

I felt a "but" coming and I soon heard her concern.

"There are a couple of things I believe about your grief. First, I think you began to grieve losing Sara about fifteen to eighteen months before she died. When you did, it changed the way you viewed your relationship. You became more caregiver and less husband. That was a huge step for you, but also a big loss. Second, when you did that, you leaped forward—sort of 'speed grieving,' moving past some things that have come back to you now that Sara has died. You need to process that before you can fully move on."

They were interesting observations and I largely agreed. Her perspective was very insightful.

As the fall of 2005 began, I stuck my toe into the dating pond. First, I went out with, oddly enough, an oncologist. We saw each other casually for a couple of months before I began seeing another woman. In one therapy session, I noted my excitement about the potential of the budding relationship, which included a decent amount of physicality, and I described it to Ann in more detail than she probably needed.

She smiled broadly and laughed before saying, "Ron, it's great to see you are starting to move on. However," she added with a laugh, "it's important to remember that you aren't seventeen anymore."

I mulled over what she said. She was right. I was approaching my new relationship life like a young man's adventure. "As you know, Sara and I were together pretty much exclusively from high school. So, I guess you're right. Maybe I'm approaching this from some long-ago, adolescent dating perspective."

She laughed again and said it was understandable. But she added that I had to process and keep that in mind as I made my way through the dating world. Take it as it comes, I thought. And if I was truly looking for a partner, I would need to get beyond the frivolous, superficial, and physical part of dating and settle into a more thoughtful and serious approach. She added she knew I'd said I was committed to that eventuality and it would come. But, she noted, I should take things slowly and be patient.

We covered lots of territory through the year I worked with her: the kids, other family dynamics, my job situation, finances, lots more about dating. Nothing was off-limits. I enjoyed our conversations and was ready to learn more about myself, as well as others in my life. Her feedback and insights were invaluable as I emerged from my depressed and lonely state.

As we concluded our sessions in the late Spring of 2006, I felt a real sense of loss. Ann had given me counsel that allowed me to move on. I considered her a friend and knew I would miss her guidance. As it had earlier in my life, therapy had lifted me up and equipped me to move to, and effectively deal with, the next chapter of my life journey.

That journey was headed toward an unforeseen speed bump.

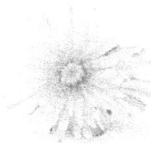

CHAPTER
19

I made my annual urology appointment in the spring of 2006. My bout with cancer and the removal of my left kidney in 2000 seemed experiences from a distant point in time. I had followed up yearly and all had been fine.

I relaxed on the exam table as the technician moved the ultrasound handset over my abdomen. My mind hazily drifted back to that November day nearly six years earlier when they discovered my kidney cancer. She completed the exam and gave me a towel. I wiped the gel from my abdomen and replaced my shirt. I went into the urologist's office and waited for what I thought was too long before he came in.

He didn't even say hello.

"Well, Ron, remember that small mass in your right kidney we saw when we did that MRI back in 2000?"

I said yes and immediately felt a knot start to grow in my stomach.

"That mass has grown into a tumor. It's very suspicious and I have to say, I'm quite certain it is cancerous."

He had always been frank and forthright and I appreciated that. But this left me speechless.

I tried to gather my thoughts, but they were caroming off one another like pinballs against bumpers. *I've already done this. This isn't supposed to happen. How unfair is this? How could this be?* I had no symptoms—no back pain or blood in my urine.

"Okay," I said as I swallowed hard and he looked me in the eye across his massive desk. It seemed he shared my disbelief. "So what's next? I suppose . . . surgery?"

He paused. I could tell he was perplexed by this. It didn't follow the normal track his cases followed.

"Yes," he said, some resignation in his voice, "and, as we did before, we should deal with this quickly."

"Yeah, unfortunately, I know the routine," I said.

"I know this doesn't make it any easier, but this is highly unusual," he said. "To have cancer in both kidneys is pretty rare."

I laughed sarcastically. "Yeah, that's a real comfort. Can't I be a rarity in some more positive way?"

We scheduled the surgery for the next week. I thought about the kids as I drove home. They had lost Sara a year ago and now they faced their dad having cancer.

I called soon after to tell Andrew, and it seemed he took it relatively well, though I could sense concern in his voice. He said he would come home for the surgery. I told Jenny after she got home from school later in the day.

"Will you be okay, Dad?" she asked, worry washing over her face. "You aren't going to die, are you?"

I could only imagine what was going on in her head. She was about to graduate from high school, had lost her mom, and now had to be wondering about losing her dad. Heavy stuff for anyone, but especially for an adopted kid with a mental illness, struggling to get her life started.

On the night before the surgery, Andrew and I talked about the procedure. I had to cover the "tough stuff" that would normally be done with a spouse. I never expected to discuss the possibility of dying with my son when in my mid-fifties.

"We've already talked about the will and how you're my medical advocate," I said to him. I had created a special needs trust that would provide for the two of them—particularly Jenny—in a measured and thoughtful manner. "I'm confident everything will go all right tomorrow, but if something goes wrong, you know that I don't want to be kept alive by artificial means, by machines or anything else."

He looked down at the floor. "I know, Dad," he said quietly. "I'd make sure they honor your wishes."

We were silent for a few moments before I responded.

"I hate that we're having this conversation, Scooze. You've gone through way too much in your young life. I'm so proud of the way you've handled it."

As is Andrew's way, he humbly dismissed his contribution. "Thanks, Dad. Will your kidney be okay? Will you need to do anything special—eat differently or take any drugs after surgery? Will there be more treatment, like radiation?"

"I don't think so," I said, reiterating what we had discussed as we first spoke on the phone. "Dr. Vora believes the tumor is in a position that will allow him to remove some of the lower portion of my kidney but leave more than half of it. He said I should have normal function and shouldn't need to do anything more."

We trouped to the hospital early the next morning. I was in surgery for more than five hours as they carved their way around the tumor, making sure I had enough kidney to let me live a normal life. In the end, it all went well. My kidney has functioned at a normal level since.

It was another moment of reckoning in our family's collective life. The kids handled it well. Sara's cancer had been our focus for so long, and now, I had my second go-round with the disease. I considered myself very fortunate; the outcome could've been far different.

I surmised there was a reason I was still around. Trying to understand it could have been mind-boggling and driven me crazy. I chose to accept it and move on.

Following the surgery, I made a vow to get serious about three aspects of my life: working to get myself into better shape; getting back into the PR and communications work world; and dating, discovering, and settling in with the woman who wanted to join me on my life journey.

I continued slogging through my work in financial services. The one thing I did enjoy was helping my clients become more comfortable with their financial situations. It was tough sledding, trying to build my business, and while using the position to gain schedule flexibility to be with Sara had worked, it had been done at the expense of my personal finances.

After all I'd been through—caring for Sara, dealing with Jenny, and my cancer—I finally admitted to myself that I didn't have enough energy—or commitment—to make my financial services business work. PR and communications were calling me, and I needed to return to the career I had left four years before.

I searched in earnest for a senior-level position in the Detroit area, but there wasn't much available. I talked with several companies and agencies but kept coming away empty. My frustration with the lack of opportunity was growing.

In early 2007, I interviewed with one of the best agencies in Detroit. All had gone well and I left the Motor City to go to a friend's wedding in California on a Thursday in February. As I stood at baggage claim at the Orange County airport, I checked my voice mail and discovered a message from one of the agency partners. He said he was pleased to extend an offer to head up the PR and marketing communications efforts on a piece of automotive business.

Finally . . . it's going to work out, I thought to myself. I had wondered if this would ever come to be.

I flew back to Detroit Sunday evening and, on Monday, I was upbeat and excited as I went to the agency for an afternoon meeting to finalize the details of my agreement. I thought about strategy related to the account on the drive over and as I waited in the conference room. The agency's two principals walked into the room and, as they entered, I could see by the expressions on their faces, all was not right.

"Ron, I'm afraid we have some news that isn't so good," said the older of the two. "The company we were expecting you to work with contacted us Saturday to let us know they're putting the account up for review."

I was stunned. This was the position that would allow me to stay in Detroit, make a decent living, and start getting back on my feet financially.

"Under those circumstances, we can't justify bringing you on board," he added. "We're sorry. You'd be such a great fit and a fantastic addition to our practice, one that would make us a stronger organization."

I didn't really hear much after that. I wanted to walk out but maintained my composure as they went on for a bit, saying how miserable this was and how badly they felt.

As I drove home, I felt like I had been kicked in the stomach. What was I going to do? I couldn't afford to continue taking a financial beating or I would have to file for bankruptcy. The anticipation of a new job had me even more checked out on my financial services practice than I had been before.

My search floundered the next few weeks. Then I headed to Denver to be with a group of longtime friends to celebrate the sixtieth birthday of Tim Simmons, who we'd visited on our Colorado trip a few years earlier. Tim's wife, Lynn, had organized a weekend-long party for him. I scrimped and saved so I could go. This was a get-together I couldn't miss.

It was a fun weekend; a terrific diversion for me as I was grappling with the job difficulties I faced. As I talked with my Colorado friends, several asked me if I had considered returning to the Rockies. They wondered why I was staying in Michigan.

Honestly, it had never dawned on me to move back to Colorado. I figured I would end up in Michigan, where family was close by. Then too, Jenny seemed to want to stay around Detroit and I thought it would be in her best interests to remain there.

But the Colorado trip piqued my interest in returning to the Rockies and I began to look at job possibilities in the Denver area. About two weeks after I returned to Troy, I saw a senior-level communications position for Covidien, a major healthcare company. A close friend, Eric Kraus, was head of communications there.

I called and asked him about the job. He told me he'd check into it and get back to me. He called later in the day and told me I had an interview in Boulder the following Tuesday. After a second interview, the company offered me the job. I couldn't believe it. I was going to return to communications and PR. I immediately began preparations for the move to the Denver suburbs. It felt, in some ways, like I was going home.

I started in July of 2007 and it was great to be back in the Rockies. The healthcare world was new for me, but I enjoyed knowing I was working in an industry that helped thousands of people worldwide—as well as their families and friends— every day. It was a great feeling of satisfaction after working for so many years in sports and the beer industry, where we put on successful, major events and entertained thousands of people. I had often wondered, though, what difference my work in sports really made in the big picture. Plus, with all the time I'd spent with Sara in the healthcare system, I had developed an interest in and decent level of understanding of the industry.

I worked at Covidien for two years before I grew weary of the company obsession with process and their demand that I focus almost exclusively on it within communications. While process is a piece of what's necessary in any position, it is not why I enjoy communications and it certainly was not why I joined the company. My creative spirit was stifled and dying. I was disinterested in Six Sigma and LEAN exercises that largely told me what I already knew. In the end, I met with my superiors and decided to leave. In a few months, I started a PR and communications practice that became a success almost overnight. I continue it to this day and realized soon after, I love working from the office at home and being my own boss. I should've done it sooner.

Leaving the corporate world I had worked in for so many years was far easier than I expected, and there was one primary reason: I had met the woman who, I knew from our very first date, was going to bring joy back to my life.

Lisa and I met on eHarmony and very quickly fell in love. It happened so fast and felt so comfortable. I'd missed a serious relationship, just as Sara had predicted. I looked forward to again enjoying the life of a married man.

The road to marriage, though, had been filled with twists and turns and several bumps along the way. About nine months after Sara died, I was dating a woman I met through work, and we saw one another for about six months before the relationship began to unravel. I had not experienced rejection for many years and it was not an easy thing for me. Since it was my first relationship after Sara died, I chalked it up to learning along the way.

There was a lot more learning for me over the next couple of years. I was quite naïve about the dating world. Sara and I had gone steady in high school, moved on to college, and, for the most part, had been together for all our adult lives. I didn't date much beyond the age of sixteen, and my lack of experience didn't serve me well, as I had discussed with my therapist, Ann, when I dove back into the dating pond.

As that first relationship wound down, I had begun to delve into the world of Internet dating. Wow! I found it to be such as easy way to meet women. So much so that, at times, it was almost scary. What an experience it was, though—particularly for a guy who had been away from dating as long as I had.

Through the end of 2006 and for the next two-plus years, I was out there in the dating world. A lot.

One evening after Lisa and I had gotten together, we were casually discussing our pasts. She asked me how many women I'd dated after Sara died.

"I don't know, I never really counted," I replied, attempting to dismiss the question.

"Was it ten? Twenty? More?" she asked.

I thought about it for a bit, calculating in my mind, and then offered an estimate.

"Probably somewhere around forty," I said.

Lisa seemed startled by the number.

"Really? That many?"

"Well, that includes women I went out with only once all the way through to a couple I saw many times over several months," I said with a laugh. "It was quite an experience. I could write a book."

As I looked back, there were a couple things that really stood out. First, how many women there were who had previously been in miserable relationships. I'd been in a great marriage, so I really had no other frame of reference. I was not so naïve that I didn't understand there was a lot of divorce and many people in bad relationships. But it really hit me as I listened to many of the women I discovered in the dating world. After hearing story after story (and, yes, I recognize there is always more than one side to a story), I have to say, there is something to the whole "guys are pigs" perspective we've all heard about. Frankly guys, aren't we better than this? Treating someone with respect, in a loving way, is really not that difficult. Then too, after a couple of my dating experiences, I have to say it applies to a handful of women, too.

Second, it amazed me how many women were interested in, shall we say, "physical" relationships. Maybe it was a reflection of a guy who grew up in a somewhat sheltered world in the '60s, but where were all the ladies I had heard wanted a "sensitive, respectful, and caring" guy? It was somewhat startling how easily things progressed.

It was a very interesting time in my life. But by the time I met Lisa, the thrill of it was long gone. I was growing weary of the dating world and was pleased to put it behind me. Lisa provided the long-term stability, commitment, and true love I craved, and, I'm so pleased to say, our relationship is one that only gets better as time passes.

I could offer many other suggestions about Internet dating, but I'll only say one more thing. Don't be surprised by *anything* you find out there. Patience and a dose of caution are very good things when you are meeting people for the first time, especially in a medium where they can appear to be something they are not. Be wary.

The other main event in my life centered around my daughter. As planned, Jenny had moved back in with me a couple of weeks after Sara died. She'd been in major psychiatric treatment and care at Havenwyck for eighteen months.

I was happy she was home and cautiously optimistic that it would work. She seemed less volatile and it appeared she had made good progress during her stay. But the proof would be in her behavior.

When Jenny returned home after Sara's death, she again attended school at the Oakland County facility that offered programs for kids with emotional and behavioral issues. She did reasonably well, finishing her junior year there. She was assigned to the school for the first semester of her senior year, but went to Troy Athens High School for her final semester and then graduated.

Beginning as a second-semester senior at Athens meant she was regularly on the outside looking in, socially. There were also a few kids who seemed determined to pick on her. Jenny had a handful of friends from her earlier years in the neighborhood and her elementary school days, but she spent much of her high school time by herself. It had to be extremely difficult for a senior struggling to insert herself into such a highly competitive and, often, catty world.

There was one instance in which her day-to-day situation came to a head. One evening, she, Andrew, and I were on our way to dinner and I asked her how her day had gone. She was unusually forthcoming in her response. Rather than the typical, "Fine," she spoke of a few girls who had been teasing her on the bus ride home and it was obvious it bothered her greatly. She broke into tears as she described it, and I felt helpless as her dad, thinking of all she had endured the past several months. It wasn't fair to have to face people who were intent on being mean to her.

As time passed, Jenny continued to do better than she had during previous home stays. She was focused on school and determined to get her high school diploma. We talked about her future and decided she would go to Oakland Community College, the local two-year school. In a perfect world, she would get a degree and transfer to a four-year school where she would probably study to become a teacher.

Not all was rosy, though. We had several moments of confrontation because Jenny, at times, exhibited behavior that was oppositional, angry and, occasionally, bizarre. One thing that was becoming apparent was her lack of judgment. She regularly struggled with relationships, often making questionable choices about friends—particularly guys—and generally found it challenging to problem-solve issues and situations.

Jenny started at Oakland and was genuinely excited about her future. She'd taken driver's education during the summer and gotten her license, giving her the independence teenagers relish. Her driving freed up time I needed to work on my struggling financial services business.

She consistently went to school, but she was having troubles with her studies. I tried to help, but I wondered if she was actually attending classes and keeping up. She assured me she was studying and I believed her—until we received her grade report at the end of the term. Her GPA was less than 1.0, and I told her she would have to do better to remain in school. I intervened to get her help at the college and encouraged her to reach out to tutors, meet with her advisors, and talk with others who could help her do better academically.

In the end, though, she was not making acceptable grades. She was allowed to start the following school year on a probationary basis. Unfortunately, the results were not much different. She ended up with only a handful of credits after her community college stint, and I was fast coming to the conclusion she was going to have to find a different direction in her life.

Then came the transition to Colorado. I accepted my job and told Jenny, who was now nineteen, that she could stay in the Detroit area if she wanted, but that I thought it would be in her best interests to join me in Colorado. It was obvious she didn't want to leave Michigan, but she relented and moved with me in August of 2007.

As is generally the case with a new, senior-level job, I was extremely busy and had little time to help Jenny. I did what I could but was trying to get my head back into a corporate mindset, learn a new industry, and get on with my life. It would have been a bumpy transition for any nineteen-year-old, but especially so for Jenny with her limitations.

She wanted to attend community college in Colorado. I told her we would give it one more shot and, if she couldn't handle it, she would have to find a job or go in a different direction. She seemed to really try, but she was often irritable and lashed out at me in ways that were hurtful and difficult to absorb. I wanted the best for her but knew we faced an uphill battle.

Finally, the decision was made for us. Her grades were not high enough for her to continue community college. She talked about going to massage therapy school and also said she was interested in cosmetology school. The latter is where she landed. She seemed to do fine with her learning but was missing classes because she was unable to get herself up and going on most mornings. Her lack of attendance came back to haunt her as she was terminated by the school.

In the interim, she and I had moved in with Lisa and her daughter, Grace, and, while we gave it all we could to make it work, it came to a head one August morning after Jenny had again battled me about getting up to go to school.

After Jenny left, Lisa and I talked about it.

"Ron, I don't know how you've done this for all these years," she said. "But we can't continue to have this go on here. We can't live like this."

The turmoil I'd experienced in living with Jenny all those years had become a way of life for me. I didn't fully realize the magnitude of the stress until someone else saw it, firsthand.

The situation had been building to a head pretty much since we moved in. Jenny's oppositional behavior grew and the tension in the house was palpable. Her anger was aimed mostly at me, and Lisa was concerned about the toll it was taking on me physically. After my bouts with cancer, we were trying to minimize the stress and other variables that might affect my health.

We thought therapy would help and convinced Jenny to attend a session with us. After fifteen minutes of discussion, she stormed out. All this, coupled with the fact I'd known for several years that Jenny was an experiential learner, led us to decide it would be best for all of us if she was on her own. We could talk all day about the consequences of her behavior, but until going through it on her own, Jenny never seemed to have a full understanding of how to take more responsibility for her life.

We found an apartment for her near the cosmetology school and she moved out of our home a couple of weeks later. She has advanced from that circumstance and, to this day, we continue to provide her some financial support and regularly talk with her about strategies that could help her to better manage her day-to-day life.

Lisa was right; I had acquiesced for too long. She was deeply concerned with the amount of stress the situation brought to my life. Making this change would help eliminate some of that.

As parents, though, it was difficult to let Jenny go out on her own, knowing how she would struggle. At twenty-five, she continues to make small increments of progress while occasionally stumbling along the way. Unlike the finite scenario experienced as Sara faded away, the ever changing world of mental illness brings with it a sadness that comes with having to regularly adjust expectations in a way I never imagined. With that said, we regularly do a re-set with Jenny, hoping to see her make better choices. She has shown glimmers of progress and, ultimately, the ball is in her court. We remain hopeful that she will pick it up and run with it in a way that will enhance her life.

AFTERWORD

Some have asked me, "Where does life go after all the adversity and turmoil? How do you go on?"

I certainly don't have all the answers. Sometimes, though, I think I should.

When I set out to tell our story, I didn't intend for it to be some sort of self-help book. As Sara was dying, she and I talked several times about sharing our experiences with the hope it would be of benefit to some. I trust, on some level, *Dodging Dandelions* does that.

As I have traveled my journey, I learned many things. One of the most important is to always be completely honest with yourself about your situation. If you don't recognize what you face, there's no way you'll ever be able to manage and effectively deal with it.

Once you've done that, you have to honestly process your emotions—the disbelief, anger, sense of unfairness, sadness, depression, and whatever else is churning inside you. All of it must be openly and genuinely considered and dealt with.

Then accept where you are. Embrace your circumstances. And make the very best of them.

Only then will you be able to move on.

It's my experience that acceptance is the most important piece of the process. It's critical to being able to move forward. There's no right or wrong in reaching your level of acceptance. By the way, reaching your level of acceptance doesn't mean you passively take what is being dished your way. You don't roll over like a submissive dog under attack. You actively do all you can to resolve the situation in the best manner possible.

What I've grown to understand, too, is that acceptance doesn't necessarily apply in the same way in every circumstance. Acceptance was crucial as I dealt with Sara's illness, and doing so allowed me to provide her with what I would characterize as a good level of care.

Unconditional acceptance does not work universally. I managed to accept where I was with Jenny and, in doing so, nudged along some resolution in a difficult situation. Acceptance, in that case, meant generating significant change and ending turmoil, becoming extremely proactive, setting better boundaries, and recognizing that I should not accept the anger and rage being directed at me. It also meant taking action that, for too long, I didn't fully understand I needed to take. In the end, all of us are better off for the changes we made. Our lives would never have moved ahead without a high level of acceptance. We've reached a working solution for a very difficult situation.

As each of us figures out, fully understands, and accepts our situation, we must decide the best way to manage it. Once done, I found it important to move on to create a well-conceived and thoughtful plan. Execute that plan with a sense of honesty, open-mindedness, flexibility, and humility. Make sure you do what's in your best interests, as well as the interests of those you hold close around you. Then accept— and own—the outcome. After doing so, move forward.

Since first learning of Sara's cancer thirty years ago, the ups and downs have been too numerous for me to count. As I said, I don't have all this figured out. But I do have a unique insight shaped by many experiences as we wound our way through the never-ending events we faced.

My thinking has always been based on a foundation of seeking and finding adventures. It is a perspective Sara and I shared, and one that has a prominent place in the relationship Lisa and I have created and developed. Within the context of that viewpoint, I am convinced that life is meant to be lived fully and vibrantly. We are not here to approach things halfheartedly. I know all too well there are moments when we have an opportunity to slack off. I was faced with that possibility often as I cared for Sara, particularly in the final years of her life. That was especially true when it was time to make a choice about serving as her primary caregiver. There were many times when it would have been easier to let things go, to not make a vigorous, concerted effort to move forward. But had I done so, I would have regrets today, and I would not have the excellent life I now have.

Lisa and I occasionally talk about when we first met and started dating. I was truly at a crossroads. I had been dating with a vengeance over the past couple of years and it was not working out as I had hoped. I had met and dated dozens of women, but none was the partner I wanted permanently in my life. I came very close to using the excuse that it was nearly a sixty-mile drive each way to see Lisa as the reason to not date her.

What a monumental mistake it would have been had I made the decision to not begin a relationship with Lisa. We met in the spring of 2009 and married a year later. After so many start-and-stop dating dalliances, I had been on the verge of stopping. Had I done so, my life would not have taken the positive turn it has with Lisa as my partner.

I genuinely hope you never experience significant losses in your life. They are times that generate pain and sadness. It's extremely important to move through the stages I have described previously, achieve acceptance, and then move on so you can again feel the joy that you deserve in your life.

One final thought. Recovery really does happen.

Loss is devastating, overwhelming, a black hole of near hopelessness and depression. For a period of time, your loss can pull you down. Talk about it with others. Allow for time to process it. Do so at your own speed. Remember, there is no right or wrong period of time to deal with it, to grieve it. At some point, though, you must accept it. Then move forward.

It reminds me of when you sit or stand in one place too long. You begin to sink. And it often feels very comfortable to settle in.

But don't settle. Don't get pulled down. Make the choice to take that step to get up. Then keep moving . . . forward.

Sara helped me understand, as Lisa does to this day, that there's a wonderful world out there for each of us. We just have to recognize it and then choose to pursue and create it.

If there's one thing that came through as you read our story, I hope it's this: Life doesn't end when adversity rears its head.

It is just then that you dodge the dandelions and turn the page to the next chapter of your journey.

ACKNOWLEDGMENTS

Dodging Dandelions was written entirely from my recollections. It's ironic in a way because, for much of my adult life, I walked around with a reporter's notebook stuffed in my left rear pants pocket. I'm confident my remembrances are accurate, although a few of the dates may not be exact. Honestly, the amount of detail I recalled twenty years after the fact was often startling.

There are many who have helped my story become reality. Melanie Mulhall is a fabulous editor and I thank her for her meaningful insights and guidance. Helena Mariposa's proofreading talents are top-notch and I am grateful for her cleansing of my copy. Nick Zelinger provided great counsel on the design and layout of Dodging Dandelions and I thank him for his forward thinking and approach. Also, I want to say a thank you to those individuals I've met through the Colorado Independent Publishers Association who have offered advice. They, too, have provided me with many useful insights.

I owe a big and loving thank you to my children, Andrew and Jenny. They gave me feedback on my writing and helped with information that filled gaps and further enhanced the story.

Finally, to Lisa, the second love of my life. I am so fortunate to have found you so we could share our journey. Your suggestions, perspective, encouragement, and support have been invaluable, and I could not have completed this work without you. You have brought the joy back to my life. I love you, Sweetie.

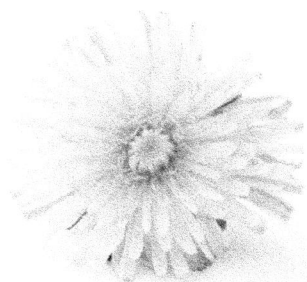

www.ingramcontent.com/pod-product-compliance
Lightning Source LLC
Chambersburg PA
CBHW021614270326
41931CB00008B/695